Unbreaking the Soul

Unbreaking the Soul

Healing with Heart-Centered Hypnotherapy

Written With Love By Jyoti Ma

Copyright© 2016 by Melody Litton, CHt

All rights reserved

www.healingforlifewa.com

For Shahn, Michael, and

Na Lamaku

I gently guide my client into hypnosis and watch as his body relaxes, moving deeper and deeper into a trance.

"Henry, tell me where you are." *I ask, after guiding him through a regression.*

"I'm at the hospital. It's March 3rd, 1967 at 11:04 AM."

"Please," *I gently invite,* "share what you're experiencing."

He responds slowly, with intense emotion, "I was just born. I came out backwards. It was so hard . . . so hard." *A single tear is dripping off the side of his left cheek.*

I witness this grown man lying in my office exuding the demeanor and meekness of an infant and encourage him to continue exploring this consciously forgotten experience from long ago.

"The doctor is telling my mother that I'm a boy." *He pauses for several minutes and when he begins again, he has to force the painful words to leave his lips.* "She says she wishes I had never been born. She says she wanted me to be a girl." *He cries openly for several moments and the tears flow like rivers from his eyes,* "She doesn't want me to be born."

"Henry, what are you feeling? Check inside your body and please share with me the strongest emotions you're experiencing."

"I'm so sad. I have a right to exist. Why is she being so mean? I'm angry. I'm hurting. I have a right to exist! I worked so hard to come. I want her to love me. I want my mommy to love me and want me!" *Uncontrolled sobbing erupts from the deepest part of his being, filling the room with a palpable energy of sorrow.* "I have the right to exist. I have the right to be born."

I allow him to cry for several minutes before encouraging him to continue exploring the memory. "During this early experience, you made a negative conclusion about yourself and it's stayed with you. What conclusion did you make?"

He immediately knows the answer but the words come as a whisper, carrying the heavy weight of shame and sadness. "I am not enough. . . I'm not enough."

Contents

Introduction 1

Chapter One: Heart-Centered Hypnotherapy 5

Chapter Two: The Highest Self 11

Chapter Three: The Body- A Window to the Soul 21

Chapter Four: Spirit Fragments 33

Chapter Five: Loved Ones and Angels 47

Chapter Six: God's Role in Healing 59

Chapter Seven: Addiction From the Inside Out 71

Chapter Eight: Our Relationship with Food 81

Chapter Nine: False Conclusions 97

Chapter Ten: Looking Within 111

Chapter Eleven: Womb and Early Life Experiences 123

Chapter Twelve: Destructive Patterns 137

Chapter Thirteen: Energetic Bonds 149

Chapter Fourteen: It's Time to Heal 167

Introduction

Everything that we have experienced stays within us. Each memory is stored and labeled inside our subconscious mind. Each experience builds upon the last. During our earliest years we form conclusions about ourselves that influence how we will act and what we expect. Some of these conclusions are positive; many are not. Because we are not consciously aware, we find ourselves repeating life patterns over and over again, never understanding why and, perhaps, losing hope that things can ever change.

We desire to be happy. We desire to feel good about ourselves. We desire to live lives with meaning and to have loved ones who love, support, appreciate, and care about us. We desire to have control of ourselves, our lives, and to create something worth having. But these things seem to continually allude us. We try and try and are too often met with failure after failure. We fail to accomplish what matters. We fail to build meaningful relationships. We fail to overcome habits or behaviors we want so badly to abandon. We fail to become the person we truly want to be. Often, we even fail to appreciate, recognize, and celebrate our successes.

Throughout this book I will share glimpses into the souls of individuals just like you and me; people who are doing the best they know how and who are ready for a happier and more fulfilling existence. I use a combination of Heart-Centered Hypnotherapy and various energy healing techniques to guide individuals in uncovering hidden sources of brokenness and pain. As understanding and awareness expand, healing begins from the inside out.

At our core, we are love and light. We are beauty, innocence, and unlimited potential. The problem is we forget. We forget the truth of who we are and begin to believe lies. As we believe lies, darkness begins to block the light and blind us from taking the life paths that lead to our greatest and happiest existence.

This book illustrates some of the ways darkness sneaks into your life, allowing the lies to take seed. It will expand your understanding of the factors that contribute to who you are and offer insight into why others are the way they are. Most importantly, it will rekindle hope that healing and positive change are not only possible, they are happening every day.

It's my hope and goal to guide as many people as I can back to the light within. As we come to understand and find the light within ourselves, it becomes much easier to see this light within others—even when it is buried deeply. As we draw upon our own light and as we call upon the light within others, we change our reality. We change the world—one soul at a time. And that change begins by opening our eyes to the truth: *We are divine, radiant beings full of love, light, and unlimited potential.*

Chapter One

Heart-Centered Hypnotherapy

"The greatest journey you will ever take is the journey within."

Hypnosis is a natural state of relaxed, focused attention. While in hypnosis, an individual is not asleep or unconscious and they do not surrender control. Hypnotherapy is the use of hypnosis with the intention of helping an individual to create positive change or to experience self-reflection. A skilled hypnotherapist is able to guide a client into the deep pockets of the subconscious mind in order to better understand themselves, their behavior, and their emotions. They can also guide the client in releasing the blocks and fears holding them back from making positive change and embracing a happy life.

Heart-Centered Hypnotherapy is a specialized and highly effective modality developed by Diane Zimberoff and is taught by The Wellness Institute, based in Issaquah, Washington. It is founded in the work of Carl Jung, Abraham Maslow, Fritz Perls, Eric Berne, Stanislav Grof, and over 15 other top psychotherapists.

I was divinely led to The Wellness Institute where I trained as a Heart-Centered Hypnotherapist. My life has never been the same.

In this book I share Heart-Centered Hypnotherapy sessions that I have been directly a part of. Most of them I facilitated as hypnotherapist, some of them I observed or supervised, and a couple of them are my own experiences as a client with another therapist guiding the session.

Each session is presented in the present tense in order for you to

Jyoti Ma • 7

easily follow along with the client's emotions and experience, just as I do while facilitating. These excerpts are shared with full permission; names and some key details have been changed in order to honor privacy and anonymity. I would like to take a moment to thank and honor each individual who willingly allowed their sessions to be shared in hopes it would make a difference in the life of another.

In a hypnotic trance, we are deeply connected to the emotions stored within our body and subconscious mind. Emotions often come up much more strongly than when in our conscious state. It's very common for someone to describe a trauma to me during the beginning of their appointment with a calm voice and without any tears. They might explain it away with statements like: "But I'm over it. I feel really OK with it now." However, once in a trance, the part of the client that is holding the pain, grief, anger, or other emotional response to the event, will often surface and the client will find themselves experiencing incredibly intense levels of emotion and speaking words and thoughts they hadn't consciously acknowledged.

Early on in life, most of us were conditioned to push down and stuff our emotions inside: "Good girls don't cry." "Quit being a baby." "Be a man. Stop whining." "You need to be strong. Don't let them see you upset." In addition to social conditioning, punishment by our parents and peers bear an impact. Shaming, corporal punishment, and physical abuse quickly teach a child that showing feelings is wrong or unsafe.

Fear, along with our desire to please, lead us to suppress our emotions. Many individuals have learned to do this so well that they don't feel at all—at least not on a conscious level. But it's all still there. And sometimes it is overwhelmingly intense. Whether we consciously acknowledge our emotions or not, they have an incredible impact on our lives. Our body, mind, and spirit are all affected by what we are storing within.

Negative emotions, along with negative subconscious beliefs about ourselves and expectations about the world, impact our lives in very real and powerful ways. Consider a beautiful lawn of grass with weeds sprouting up in various places. If we were to simply break off or cut the weeds down, they would continue to grow back and affect the health and quality of the lawn. If, however, we dig down and find the root, the weed can be removed for good.

This is the intention of Heart-Centered Hypnotherapy, to find the deepest roots of misunderstanding and false beliefs in order to remove them for good. Once the root is gone, other pieces and fragments of the weed will wither and die much more readily, allowing the soul to heal. This does not mean that our earliest experiences are the only ones that matter or affect us. It does mean that our earliest experiences form the deepest roots. Future beliefs and negative conclusions are added to and grown from these early seeds of pain and misunderstanding. When we heal the deepest parts of our self, every part of us is affected for the better.

This may be a new concept for you and I encourage you to simply allow my words to gently plant a healthy seed. This seed of understanding and awareness will grow as you continue to read and meditate on the words and stories shared within this book. I encourage you to be mindful of your emotions and even physical responses as you read. Journal the feelings and memories that surface. Meditate on the impressions that come or explore them with the help of a Heart-Centered Hypnotherapist.

Chapter Two

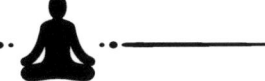

The Highest Self

*"When you stop looking outside of yourself for answers,
and instead look within, you will discover
a wealth of knowledge and an abundance of peace."*

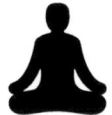

One of the most important goals that I have for clients is to help them reconnect with their Highest Self. Other professionals may refer to the Highest Self in various terms; the Authentic Self, the Wise Adult, the Inner Light, the True Self, or the Superconscious. My preferred term is Highest Self as I feel it best represents the nature of this divine part within us.

The Highest Self is the part of us who sees clearly. It's the part of us who is wise and isn't controlled by negative emotion and whose judgment is never clouded by false beliefs. The Highest Self is the eternal part of our being, the brightest part of our soul. It's the part who has always existed and will always exist. It has an understanding of our life purpose and a road map guiding us in that purpose. The Highest Self is directly connected to God, to the light of truth, wisdom, knowledge, and, most especially, love.

The Highest Self steps in, as often as we allow, to help and guide us. It is the gentle whisper of wisdom and confidence we need in the midst of discouragement and fear. It's the love that rises to the surface when hate or anger could be the alternative. It's the courage we find when we have difficult decisions to make. It's the wind that gently blows us in one direction when we thought our life was headed in another.

The Highest Self is the purest part of our being. It is the part that remains beautiful even when the rest of us is weighed down by darkness or pain. The existence of the Highest Self teaches me that no one is beyond saving and no one is beyond healing or growth. Everyone, with help and love, can kindle this light within and find root again in truth and peace no matter what they've been through.

Whenever possible, I strive to help clients begin connecting with the Highest Self from the very beginning of their healing journey. The Highest Self will then guide all healing, in the right time and in the way that serves the client's highest good. At times, the disconnect between the individual and their Highest Self is so severe that reconnecting is impossible in the beginning. But with time and loving patience, this connection can occur and is vital to lifelong healing and positive growth.

The following excerpts will help you begin to understand the Highest Self and the important role it plays.

Note: The examples I share within each chapter are relevant excerpts from sessions and do not represent everything that took place. Care was taken to create a feeling of safety for each client and sufficient time granted to guide them into a proper level of trance. Some clients needed several sessions before they were ready to address core issues. Others, their first time in hypnosis, were able to move quickly back to the deepest roots.

Raja, age 26, is a single mother of a 2-year-old son. Recently divorced, she is trying her best to get her life together, to be there for her child, and to find peace. In her pre-session interview, she expressed the following: "I don't feel worth very much. Nothing turns out good and I am stressed all the time."

Hypnotherapist: I invite you to go somewhere very safe, somewhere you enjoy being and can relax. Find yourself using all your senses to be there, breathing in the colors, textures, sounds, and smells.

Raja (R): I'm outside by a lake. There are beautiful flowers, green grass. It's so peaceful.

Raja, within you there is a wise adult. This is your Highest Self. It's the part of you that is healthy and directly connected to God. She is eternal, in control, and calm. She can clearly see the path ahead; she knows where you have been and where you are headed. At times throughout your life she has stepped in to guide and help you. As we begin acknowledging her, I ask her to guide you to a time or experience in your life where she was fully present, where she stepped in to help you make a healthy or good choice in your life.

R: When I lived in Connecticut and my sister asked me to move to Florida, I trusted her. I pushed aside all my fears and left the negative environment I was in. It felt so good. It was such a healthy decision.

Beautiful. I invite you now to be guided to one more time in your life when this Highest Self stepped in to guide and help you, perhaps even an earlier time.

R: I'm a teenager. I felt so alone and sad, but then I was able to reach

Jyoti Ma • 15

out to another girl and smile. We became friends. And she introduced me to her friends. I went from being alone to having an entire group of healthy friends.

And now, Raja, I invite her to show herself to you. Visualize and invite the image of your Highest Self to come forward so you can see her. Once you see, sense, or feel her in some way, please describe it to me.

R: She's smiling at me. She's full of light. She is so beautiful. Wow. She really is beautiful. She looks like me but stands taller. Her hair is longer and flowing. She's wearing white; it's like a robe but very flowing, almost a dress maybe.

What do you see radiating from her? What qualities do you know she has?

R: She is calm. She is wise. She's at peace; her face shows so much peace. She radiates a beautiful light—it feels like love. Yes, she is radiating a pure, beautiful love. She is funny and happy and isn't stressed about anything.

Raja, I'm grateful to your Highest Self for showing you these experiences. I want you to understand now that she is a part of you. Her wisdom and strength are available to you always as you choose to reach out, ask for it, and accept it. It's already within you. Look at her and she will smile to acknowledge that what I'm saying is true. *(We spend some time deepening her connection to her Highest Self and anchoring her to peace and confidence before moving on)*

When you feel unsure, afraid, or have a decision to make, simply make your anchor. You will feel connected again to the wisdom and strength of your Highest Self. She will help you and guide you as you learn to trust her. Before we end today, I'd like to ask her if she has any words or counsel she'd like to give you.

R: *(A tear forms in her left eye and drips down her face)* She wants me to know I am safe. She's with me and I'm not alone. She wants me to know I am worthwhile, that my life has purpose and meaning. And that she will help me accomplish all I am meant to. *(The tears flowing freely now)* She says I am a good person; that I am worthy of life and love. I'm going to be ok. And so is my son.

Regina, age 20, is in a fairly new relationship with a man twenty years older than she is. Their relationship began in a strip club, she was often his dancer. He asked her to quit and she moved in with him. He bought her hypnotherapy sessions in hopes of helping her with her low self-esteem.

Regina, it looks like you're feeling something. Will you share with me what you're feeling?

R: I'm scared. I'm so scared. *(Her hands come to her face and she cups her face as if trying to hide)* I'm about 13 and I'm at a department store. My stepmom's brother brought me here. But he's been watching me. He makes me feel so gross. I . . . I am scared of him.

What's happening now?

R: He's asking me what it would take for me to sleep with him. He wants me to tell him what I'll give him. *(She starts to cough, her throat closing off even saying the words)* I can't trust anybody. There is no one I can trust.

Find yourself moving back now. Follow that belief back to an earlier time in your life when these same difficult feelings are present. *(I help her regress and move deeper into her trance)*

R: I'm 7. We're moving. I feel so much sadness. My heart is hurting so badly. My mom is here, but I can't talk to her.

What do you want your mom to know?

R: Mom, I'm so sad. I'm sad we have to start over. I'm sad everything has to change. I don't even know if you care. You don't understand.

It's not fair! I can't connect with anybody anymore. You've made it hard to trust people. You told me we would stay here and now you're making me leave.

What are you deciding about your life here?

R: I can't trust anybody. I don't want to allow anybody in.

Did this belief come now, or did it come earlier? *(She indicates earlier)* **Go there now. Gently find your way back.**

R: I see my dad. I don't know how old I am or where we are, but I see his face.

What words and pain have you been holding?

R: Dad, it makes me sad you didn't think I'm your kid. I'm sad that you've not been in my life. *(The tears are flowing and her voice is shaking)* I need you. It's not fair you have six other children with other women. You're part of the reason I can't trust anyone. You've never taught me anything. You've never shown me what I should look for in a man. You've never shown me what love is. I don't even know what love is.

Regina, what do you believe about yourself?

R: I am not important. I close myself off and choose anger instead of love. I understand anger. I don't know love. Others will always let me down. I'm on my own.

How are these early beliefs and experiences still affecting your life? Allow only your Highest Self to answer, to help you see.

R: I've been seeking love without knowing what I'm looking for. I never should have danced. It has hurt my spirit even more. I can't trust others and I can't trust myself. I believe I'll always be alone and so I continue to push others away and find ways to end relationships. One part of me is longing for connection and another part of me fears it more than anything.

Regina, I invite you to see this child, the child inside of you who is hurting so badly.

R: She's skinny and fragile. She's not smiling. She looks hopeless and sad.

Take her by the hand and guide her back to your safe and beautiful place. Show her there is beauty available to her. Guide her out of the pain and darkness she is in. Then tell her the true things she needs to hear. *(I help Regina align with her Highest Self before speaking to the hurting child)*

R: I love you. I will never leave you. Everything will be ok. I won't ever give up on you. You are beautiful and smart. Be anything you want to be. I love you so much and am always here. People make mistakes. They aren't perfect. Trust God. He'll never let you down, even when others do. You are important. Don't close yourself off. Love everybody. God put you on this earth for a reason and one day you will impact someone's life for good. I love you and God loves you. You are loved. As you choose to recognize this love, you will be able to seek love in ways that will be rewarding and beautiful in your life.

Regina, what do you know to be true?

R: I am important. I am loved.

Please spend the duration of your session being guided by your Highest Self. She will show you how these new conclusions can affect and change your life for good. Allow the music to flow through you and continue to heal so many wounds of the past. Make room within you for an understanding of love and let that love find a place deep within you. *(She lies quietly, with tears brimming as the songs play)*

R: I'm ready to create a beautiful life and to release the pain of the past. I choose to live in the Light and I know what real love is.

Chapter Three

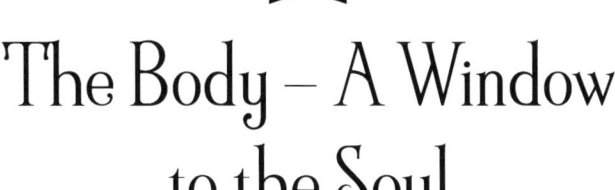

The Body – A Window to the Soul

"Listen to your body. It is your dearest friend."

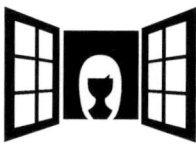

We are not only physical beings. We are also spiritual and emotional beings. These three areas must be in harmony to enjoy our greatest health and vitality. When one aspect is out of balance or in chaos, so are the others. There have been many books and extensive research completed on this mind-body connection. If you pause and pay attention, you'll recognize it within yourself.

Remember a time when you told a lie. What happened in your body when you were facing being discovered? Knots in your stomach? Sweating? And what about when your first lover said goodbye? Did you feel your heart had been torn out? You literally felt the physical crushing pain in your chest. Or perhaps when your best friend spread a rumor about you back in high school, do you remember physically feeling the blow to your gut? Have you ever been so afraid that you couldn't move, or even breathe? Our body is directly connected to our mind and spirit—each part relies upon the others to maintain and achieve our greatest health and vitality.

We use sayings all the time to explain this mind-body connection. For example, "She died of a broken heart." "He's worrying himself sick." "His cheating is driving her to the grave." "He couldn't take the stress and passed out." We recognize it with our words but often fail to see the depth and reality of the connection. We've been taught to treat our physical pain and disease with Western medicine and procedures; to treat the symptoms or to mask the root issue with pain medications or other prescription drugs. I believe that sometimes Western medicine is the answer and that medicines and surgeries can be a wonderful gift from a loving God. But I also know that all too often these methods are not needed. What's truly needed is healing within. Healing our mind and spirit leads to healing within the physical body. Disease can also be written "dis-ease"; meaning a lack of ease within the soul.

Our bodies love and serve us the best they know how. They are our companion for this life journey. Our body will carry the weight of any burden we do not choose to release in a healthy way. Every negative emotion we stuff inside, each traumatic experience that isn't processed and released, every false belief about ourselves and negative thought we hold on to has to go somewhere. Our body is that somewhere. And it holds it for us, often for years before it finally begins to show symptoms of weakening. Pain within the body often means a part of our soul needs help or that some part of us is begging for attention and healing. I'll share the story of my colleague whose experience beautifully illustrates this concept.

Through The Wellness Institute, I was allowed the opportunity to participate in their two-year advanced hypnotherapy training. As a group we learned so much; we also received incredible amounts of personal growth and healing along the way. It was such a wonderful experience to witness each individual in my group grow into their role as a healer and to see the beautiful personal transitions we each made. My colleague entered the first weekend retreat suffering severe symptoms of multiple sclerosis. She could sit with us in our learning circles for only short amounts of time. Her body ached and hurt so badly she would wear only the softest and most loosely fitting clothing. She had to request a bedroom change as the stairs were too much for her to handle. Fast forward to today. She is 65 pounds lighter, both physically and emotionally. She dresses beautifully and in well-fitted clothing. She sits with us in our meditation and learning circles for long periods of time without suffering the pain she once did. When I look at her, I see a miracle. Her smile is much brighter and the light of her aura easily fills a room. As she has learned to release the pain and emotional trauma of the past, she has allowed herself to heal and grow in truly amazing ways.

The following session excerpts will give you another glimmer of insight into this mind-body connection. The underlying factors are typically impossible to figure out with our rational mind. But once we tap into our deeper mind and follow the emotional trail, the reasons beneath the pain and dis-ease often become quite clear.

....

Kurt, age 37, owns a small business with a handful of employees. He claims to care about his employees but believes that they hate him and think he's a jerk. His lower back is constantly in pain.

....

Kurt, breathe into your lower back now. Let the physical pain that you so often experience come up in full force. Breathe and allow yourself to connect with this pain in your lower back. Once you feel it, please rate it on a scale of one to ten.

K: It's about an 8. It's a really deep aching feeling.

The answers will simply come, allow the answers to flow into your mind as I ask you questions. If your lower back had an emotion, what would it be?

K: *(He breathes and pauses for a moment. Then with surprise he answers)* Loneliness. It's lonely. And sad.

And if your back had a voice, what would it say? What words and feelings is it storing for you?

K: *(He at first shakes his head)* I don't know. *(But after a moment, words simply begin to flow out)* I'm so sad that I'm alone all of the time. I feel scared and alone all of the time. I have no one. *(The tears begin to flow and his voice begins to shake)* I try so hard and I do it all on my own. No one sees me. No one knows how hard I work. No one tries to help me. I have no support. I have no one. I am so lonely. *(Deep sobbing now)*

Now we're going to follow these emotions back. Gently find yourself going back to the source; without any effort, simply find yourself there.

K: I don't want to be alone! *(Shouting loudly)* I want my mama! *(The sobbing continues and he stops talking)*

Where are you now, Kurt?

K: I'm 15. I'm at my grandparents' house. My dad died. My mom left with her boyfriend. She left me. I cry every night. I cry uncontrollably. But I can't let anyone see. I'm too old to cry. My grandparents don't need to see me hurting like this.

This session is a time to release yourself from judgment and simply feel. Allow yourself to now express the feelings that you worked so hard to bury.

K: Mom, I don't want to be alone! *(Yelling again, deep pain in his voice)* I need to be with you. I need to know I'm loved! I'm so sad you don't want to be with me. *(The yelling stops and he continues with the meek voice of a broken child)* I'll never be happy again. I love you. But I must be unlovable. You left me. This hurts so much, Mom. I can't do this. I can't stand this.

What conclusions did you make about yourself here?

K: I am unlovable. I am going to keep everyone out. Letting people love me hurts too much because they leave and they can't love me back. I'm unsupported and on my own.

Kurt, you can begin healing this child part of yourself today. You can begin releasing the deep pain you've been carrying in your back. Would you like to do this? (He nods) OK, then please follow my lead as we walk through a process of forgiveness and release.

K: Mom, I forgive you for not being there. I forgive you for being on drugs. I forgive you for hurting me and not caring about how your actions affected me. *(Tears are flowing freely)* I forgive you for running away with a very bad man. I forgive you for abandoning me. I forgive you for not being the mom I needed. I forgive you for *(he pauses)* not loving me. *(He suddenly stops and then whispers)* I see my mom. She's here.

That's good that she's here. But I need you to notice and tell me if she looks dark or light.

K: She's dark. She's sad. *(Then turning his attention back to this image of his mother)* Mom, I forgive you. You don't need to be sad anymore. I don't want you to be sad. I don't want you to be dark. It's OK. We can both be OK. *(He begins sobbing deeply, his entire body shaking with his tears. It's several minutes before he's ready to speak again.)* She's so sorry. She's holding me and stroking my hair. She wants me to know that she does love me—that she's always loved me. She is so happy to know I've forgiven her. She's been waiting to move into the light, not wanting to leave me and feeling ashamed and unworthy. She's OK now. My grandfather is coming to take her somewhere she can be healed by the Light. She wants me to live in the Light as well.

Kurt, what does she want you to know is true about yourself? What new conclusion can you claim today?

K: I am perfect, whole, and complete. I am lovable. I am safe. I am supported in all that I do, even though that support may be invisible at times.

Kurt continued to come in for sessions regularly for a few months. He reported that the pain in his back improved dramatically as he continued to heal emotionally. He also reported feeling much more connected with his employees.

Pat, age 60, teaches at her local community college. She feels tired much of the time and also has a long standing aching pain in her right knee and is considering surgery. The pain is beginning to interfere with her ability to function and do her job.

Pat, I see emotions beginning to rise to the surface. I'd invite you to say aloud what you're feeling.

P: I'm afraid. I'm afraid I'll fail. I'm afraid if I have this knee surgery I won't heal, that I'll break. I'm afraid the new knee won't be strong enough.

I'd invite you to speak directly to your knee. What would you like your knee to know?

P: I'm sorry this happened. I could've made a choice and not been on this path. I dropped to the asphalt. This is all my fault *(tears begin to flow and her breathing shakes).*

Find yourself going back now. Simply be back in the experience you're referring to.

P: I'm going too fast! I don't know what to do. I see the gravel and the bushes and I don't want to fall. *(Gasps as she feels the fear and panic)* I'm on roller blades. Oh I'm going down. I hit hard; so hard. *(Tears continue to flow and sadness is thick in her voice)* I'm so stupid! I've made a mistake and I am so stupid. I should be walking. I shouldn't be on skates. This is all my fault. I deserve to be punished.

Pat, I want you to notice what happened when you fell and judged yourself so harshly.

P: *(Surprised)* A piece of my kneecap broke off. I see it. It's a white, clean, round ball of beautiful energy. I believe it's a piece of my self-worth, self-confidence. *(Her voice is gentle as she recognizes this part of herself and sad as she realizes it was left behind in the dirt that day)*

When this part of you broke off, what came to take its place? Breathe into your knee now and find the energy that is there.

P: It's a black mass *(pauses to tune into what she is seeing and feeling)*. It's anger and frustration. It's fear. Oh, it hurts. It makes me heavy. It reminds me of my mistakes and failures. It gives me pain. Pain is my humiliating reminder of my failure.

In order to begin the process of healing, it's important to release the harsh judgments of yourself and to extend forgiveness to yourself for this event. Is this something you feel willing to do?

P: I would like to try.

I invite you to move back into a place that feels safe, somewhere you can connect with your Highest Self and feel peace. Simply find yourself moving there now.

P: I'm on a hillside trail at Flaming Geyser. It's so beautiful. There's a wonderful light. I feel its warmth and strength. *(A beautiful energy of peace begins to wash over her)*

I'm glad you've found your way into this Light. As you extend forgiveness to yourself, you will feel this Light carrying away the darkness and pain. Speak words of forgiveness and then breathe deeply and witness this change within your knee.

P: I forgive myself for falling. I forgive myself for making a mistake. *(Speaking slowly but with sincerity)* I forgive myself for getting hurt. Accidents happen. I wasn't doing anything wrong. I forgive myself for landing on the asphalt. *(Pauses and continues with new confidence in her voice)* I choose to let go of the fear and anger. I choose to let go of this black mass of energy I've held in my knee and allow the Light to heal me. I am not stupid. I was enjoying myself and having fun. Having fun is OK and sometimes accidents happen and it's OK. I don't need to be punished for them.

Breathe out the darkness and inhale the healing Light. Then share with me what you've experienced.

P: The Light has cleansed me; the dark mass is gone. I'm inviting back the beautiful piece that broke off. It will be able to heal now; I don't need to be afraid.

As you bring back this piece of yourself, what are you reclaiming?

P: This piece was touched by the Light. As I bring it back I am given health, strength, and life. *(Pauses)* I am strong. I am focused.

In another session, Pat continued to communicate love to her knee and found other various pieces and fragments that needed healing and recognition. The knee asked her to be gentle with it and to learn to say "No" when she knew her body needed rest. She agreed to do so. She was able to successfully complete her teaching semester before having her knee surgery. Her surgery went very well and she has been quite pleased with her rate of recovery.

Pat's experience helps illustrate a very important truth. Forgiveness and self-love lead to greater healing for body, mind, and spirit. When we hold anger, resentment, harsh judgment and feelings of failure, we rob our body of its fullest ability to heal. Longstanding physical pain is often a sign that forgiveness is needed; whether toward our self or toward another.

When I do something not so smart (such as burning myself on the pan when cooking oatmeal the other morning) I immediately remember to express forgiveness to myself and then send loving thoughts to that particular part of my body. Healing comes much more quickly when we invite positive energy and love to stay with us. I invite you to begin this pattern of self-love and self-care. Be quick to forgive; decide right now to release the tendency to judge yourself or others too harshly.

Chapter Four

Spirit Fragments

*"When you feel broken and empty, don't despair.
Every scattered fragment of your soul has left a trail
to be followed when the time is right for healing."*

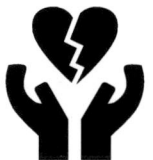

Being human is tough. Life can be awesome and wonderful; but, no matter how amazing your life may be, it's not been free of pain. No one's life is completely free of pain. For many of us, this pain has not been in short supply. Consequently, we learn to adapt; we adapt in order to survive. As you saw in Pat's experience in the previous chapter, adapting often means losing pieces of ourselves along the way. I refer to these pieces as spirit fragments.

The best way to begin understanding spirit fragments is to read the experiences of others. As you do, something will likely resonate within you, reminding you of pieces of yourself that may be lost or left behind. Many individuals speak of feeling empty or feeling unwhole. That is because they literally are.

Just a few days ago I was assisting a session with a beautiful middle-aged woman struggling with depression and an overwhelming feeling of being sucked into darkness. She regressed to age 7, the evening before her first Holy Communion. Her godfather passed away on that very night and she was left facing the events of the next day without him. Her grief was so overwhelmingly large that, as she looked into a picture of herself and her godfather, a large portion of the energy within her heart broke off and was deposited into the picture. She was able to name these fragments of herself as her hope, faith, and security. There was now a void where these feelings once resided. She described the void as a black hole. This black hole was so vast and so deep that she felt completely lost in darkness and pain. Throughout her life, this black hole continued to play a role, regularly dragging her back into darkness. It was beyond beautiful to bear witness as she found a tiny sliver of light to follow. This light guided her to these lost pieces and she was then able to invite back her hope, faith, and security.

For some, so much of the spirit has fragmented that they become merely a shell of what they once were. For others, the fragmented pieces may be quite small, representing qualities or truths they felt they needed to abandon for some reason. All of us are broken, some more than others, and each one of us needs healing. We need to retrieve pieces we have lost, and then clean, heal, and restore them, in order to be whole.

I will share a few other examples. The examples are endless as every client comes missing fragments, but in these next few pages your heart and mind will begin to see and understand the reality and implications of spirit fragments.

Jacki, age 24, came in feeling anxious. She expressed that she lives in a constant state of anxiety and sadness. She shared that, no matter how hard she tries, she always feels incapable and unworthy. She believes she's failing in every area of her life.

Jacki, find the feeling of sadness in your body. You're storing the energy of sadness and anxiety within your body. Simply breathe and ask your body to show you where it is.

J: It's in my stomach. It's so tight. It feels like it's twisting and turning around and around. It's heavy and yucky.

I invite you to breathe into that energy in your stomach now. Without any effort, simply allow the feeling or emotion found there to become very clear. What core emotion is in your stomach?

J: Sadness.

Express that sadness in words.

J: I'm sad that I don't feel like I'm doing a good job with my son. I'm sad that I don't know what I'm doing with my life. I'm sad that I won't be able to figure out what to do or even be able to do those things if I do figure it out.

Thank you for expressing this, Jacki. I invite you to explore the other emotions in your stomach now. With the sadness, there may be other feelings. Please name any other feelings.

J: There's so much sadness. *(Gently crying now)* But you're right. There's also fear. There's a lot of fear. It's overwhelming.

We're going to follow these emotions back now, back to an earlier time in your life where you felt them. We'll be moving back to the source of these feelings of fear and sadness in your life. *(I help her regress to a very early experience in her life)* **Where are you now?**

J: *(She has become very still and quiet. When she speaks, it's in a whisper)* I don't know where I am. I just feel so much pain. I am so sad and afraid.

Are you still feeling these things in your stomach?

J: Yes. It feels like too much. I don't want to feel this.

Jacki, the best way to release the pain is to express it, to honor the parts of you that are hurting by letting them talk. I invite you to breathe into your stomach and to allow the words to come, the words that have been stuck inside, churning and causing more pain.

J: I'm afraid I'm not good enough. I'm afraid I won't ever be good enough. I'll never be loved for who I am. I'll always have to be someone else in order to be loved.

What person is coming into your mind as you express these feelings?

J: My dad. *(Gentle crying is quickly becoming deep sobbing)* I've never been enough for him.

Jacki, I encourage you to speak directly to your father. Express to him these feelings you're holding inside. It's OK. It's OK to feel these things and to express them. You're safe to feel and express these things.

J: Dad, I'm afraid you'll never love me for who I am. I'm afraid I'll never be good enough for you. I'm sad that I don't feel love and acceptance from you. I'm sad that I can't be myself. *(Her voice begins rising, emotions coming even stronger now)* And I'm angry, Dad. I'm so angry. I'm angry that you made me feel this way! I'm angry that you made me feel I have to be perfect in order to be loved. I'm scared that I'm still mad at you. I'm scared that I can't move on. I'm scared that I'll pass these feelings on to my son. *(Deep sobbing, so many tears falling quickly)*

Jacki, early in your life you made a negative conclusion about yourself. What conclusion did you make?

J: I am worthless. I must do what other people want me to do so they'll like me and care about me.

(We spent the next hour visiting other times throughout her life when this negative conclusion impacted her life again and again—in school, friendships, relationships, and even now in her marriage and as a mother)

Jacki, it's time to let go of the old conclusion. It's time to release lies and to embrace truth. As you choose to release the pain, darkness, and old conclusions, you will be guided toward a happier and more fulfilling life. Is this something you feel ready to do?

J: I want to.

Then I invite your Highest Self to join you. I invite her to come to be with the little girl within you, the one who decided she was worthless and had to do what other people wanted her to in order to be accepted. Breathe and clasp your hands. Feel this wise adult joining you. What does this wise adult want this little girl to know? Allow her to be the nurturing, loving parent this little girl has been needing.

J: *(With lots of tenderness in her voice, she begins to express the words of the Highest Self to the little girl)* I love you just the way you are. You are kind and caring. You care about other people. You do your best to help others and to be happy. You love your family. You are a strong person and you can do hard things. You can accomplish things. You are important. You have people who love you for who you are. Your father did the best he knew how and in his heart he's always loved you and accepted you. It's OK to forgive him, to love him for doing his best. You have a God in your life who loves you too. You are so important to Him and He cherishes you.

Jacki, this little girl believes she is worthless and she needs to be someone different to please others and to receive acceptance. What do you want her to know instead?

J: Little one, you are precious. You are worthy of all good things. I love you and need your innocence and beauty.

I invite the Light to wash over both of you, your Adult Self and this little girl. The Light will cleanse and heal the wounds of the past and help remove the darkness and pain you've been holding in your stomach. Tell me when you can sense this.

J: I see the light. *(Tears streaming steadily)* I feel the light entering my body. It feels so warm. It's so nice. I feel so much love radiating from it.

Jackie, do you see the little girl? *(She nods)* **Is she clean and bright now?** *(She nods again)* **Is it the right time to invite her back into your body?** *(One more nod. This one is accompanied by a huge smile)*

J: Please come back. I need you. *(She reaches out as though she is taking the hands of the little girl)*

As her energy rejoins your body, mind, and spirit, what are you reclaiming into your life?

J: I am reclaiming innocence. I am reclaiming confidence. I am reclaiming the ability to love myself.

We closed the session with gentle music, allowing her energy time to balance as this wounded part of her was healed and found its way back where it belongs within her.

Annie, age 32, has a successful career and is well educated. She expressed to me that she's starting to feel a lot of bitterness and resentment toward family and friends and is unhappy with how she's been feeling. She comes from a home with a drug addicted mother and a father who was often physically, and always emotionally, absent.

Annie, I invite you to breathe deeply and simply notice what's happening within your body. Notice tightness and tension. Feel your breath moving through your body and notice where it feels blocked or clogged. *(Within minutes, Annie begins sobbing. Her tears are streaming steadily down her cheeks as she lies on the mat)* **Annie, express to me what you're feeling.**

A: I don't belong. I feel alone. I feel scared. I'm scared that I don't know what to do. I'm scared I am going to turn into someone I don't like. I hate this bitterness. I hate the anger. It feels so deep inside of me. *(The crying increases, the sobbing is getting louder)*

Without any effort, feel yourself moving to another time and place. Feel yourself in this earlier time in your life when these feelings were equally strong.

A: I cry a lot. Sometimes I cry until I pass out. I'm so little. My parents never even see me. It's like I'm here but they don't see me. I feel so alone. I cry and cry. They just ignore me. They don't care.

Speak to them now, Annie. Allow all words and feelings to simply flow from your body and through your mouth.

A: I'm here! Just see me! I matter too! *(Yelling loudly now; crying and gasping between breaths)* I know what I'm talking about. I know stuff even though you don't think I do. Please, Mom, just see me. Please, Dad, act like I matter. Please, just please be glad I'm here. *(The words stop and there are just tears, her breath still shaking)*

What conclusion did you draw about yourself here, when you were so very young?

A: I am invisible. It's better not to feel anything. My feelings are wrong. I have no reason to feel what I feel. I have to be good. If I am good then I am loved.

And what does it mean to be good?

A: To be good means to not need anything, to do what I'm supposed to do, and to not stir up any trouble.

How is this still true in your life now, your adult life?

A: No one sees me, I'm still invisible. I have to pretend all of the time. I am so very tired of pretending *(The tears are streaming still, but more gently now. An overwhelmingly hopeless feeling has entered the session)* I have to be good. I can't have needs. I have to constantly please others instead of myself.

Annie, I'm really proud of you for allowing yourself to see and feel these hard things. I'm proud of you for surviving, even though it's been so hard. I want you to know you're not alone. Notice now that you're in a beautiful meadow. Breathe and give yourself time to connect with this place, all the colors and sounds and beauty.

A: I see it. It's beautiful. There are flowers everywhere. The sky is a really bright and beautiful blue.

Now look to the outskirts of the meadow, where it meets the trees. Tell me who or what you see.

A: *(Surprise in her voice)* I see me. But it's not me. It looks like me but older. *(Long pause while she comes to understand what she's seeing)* She's an older me—the woman I want to be. She's whole. She's not angry.

Invite her to come closer. As she does, describe for me the qualities you sense radiating from her.

A: She's patient. She's at peace. She radiates this amazing love. She's smiling at me and she's so beautiful. Wait, I see someone else. It's me as a little girl. The little girl is walking toward this older me. They are both smiling now. The little girl is happy to not be alone. The older self wants me and the little girl to follow her to the river.

Go ahead. You can trust her.

A: She's washing us. She's calling down this beautiful light to touch the water and when the water touches us, it feels so warm.

Annie, what is being washed away? What are you choosing to release today?

A: I'm releasing all the pain. I am releasing shame and guilt. I feel so much weight leaving my body. The water is taking it away so easily. The light seems to linger inside my body. It's so warm. I feel so good.

This little girl, is she being washed as well? *(She nods)* **Where in your body does she belong? Where did she come from?**

A: My heart.

Would you like to welcome her back into your heart now?

A: *(With one tear)* Yes. I would. *(She reaches out and invites the girl back and then places her hands on her heart)*

What are you reclaiming as this little girl's energy finds its way back into your heart?

A: My identity. I am intuitive and sensitive to others. I am forgiving. I don't have to be afraid. I am not responsible for anyone else. I am patience and love. I can also call on this beautiful, older part of myself when I need confidence and faith.

Is it OK to be seen? Is it alright for you to have needs?

Jyoti Ma

A: Ha, yes! The beautiful woman is spreading this bright, yellow light all around me and through me. She says it's time to shine. It's time to be seen. And it's time to do the things that bring me joy.

Beautiful, Annie. Allow this yellow light to continue finding its way through you. Then see yourself shining. Shine this light to all those near and far. Claim the right to be seen and the privilege of sharing this beautiful light with all those around you.

Teresa, age 37, came in desiring to understand her need to constantly compare herself to others and feelings of inadequacy.

(After an induction and some exploration she regresses to elementary school)

T: I'm being rebellious. We're supposed to wear comfortable clothes so we can participate in PE testing. I don't want to. I chose to wear a skirt. I'm so embarrassed. I'm struggling between what I'm supposed to do and what I want to do. I feel like a fool doing testing in my skirt.

(Next regression, same year of school)

T: We're playing dodge ball. There's only me and one boy left. I lost. I let my team down. I'm disappointed and embarrassed.

What conclusions did you draw about yourself or early decisions did you make about your behavior?

T: I'm a fool. Adults have power over me. I'm not OK with them looking at me. I don't want to go against the norm anymore. I'm not going to allow myself to be the center of attention anymore.

(After some energy release and processing, she is ready to enter the healing portion of the session)

Teresa, we need to go back to the experiences you had in elementary school. Look around and something there will represent a piece of yourself that broke away from you and is still there. Take your time; it may look like you or it may be a shimmering light. Just patiently look around until you see something that you know is a part of yourself.

T: I see it. It's like a big mass. I can feel a large mass now on my chest; still separate from me.

What does this mass represent? What part of you was lost in these early experiences?

T: *(Long pause)* Confidence. It's my confidence.

(After cleansing this part of herself she was able to reconnect with it and invite it back into herself; restoring this part of her that had been broken so early in life)

T: I am a Child of God. I forgive and release these burdens. I am good simply by being myself and am now free to be exactly who I choose to be with confidence and acceptance.

Chapter Five

Loved Ones
and Angels

*"Unseen hands are holding you.
Breathe and you will feel them."*

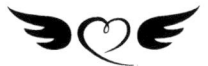

Spiritual experiences are incredibly common during Heart-Centered Hypnotherapy sessions. Whenever we seek healing, there are loved ones and angels who are waiting to assist us.

Often, the Highest Self steps forward to guide and assist the inner child and broken spirit fragments in healing. In many cases the Highest Self will be the only one to come forward to assist, but not always. Our mind and spirit know what is best and what will lead us to the greatest healing. When it's in our best interest, other angels or loved ones may also choose to come forward to help.

Deceased loved ones and even young children who have passed will often come forward. Parents and grandparents appear frequently. In other sessions, it may be aunts or uncles, cousins or friends who choose to participate in the healing. Occasionally, it's the energy of someone who is still alive. Just the other day I had a woman break down in tears when her husband's Highest Self showed up to hold her during a very painful moment in her session. They had been struggling in their marriage and he was the last person she expected to see come forward when I invited her to look. Physically living or deceased, the energy of a soul can and will show up when it's needed or when there is a higher purpose to be served. Remember, energy has no boundaries and is not limited by time or space.

While facilitating a session, when I feel the energy shift I simply ask them who has come to be with them. Without fail, the client either knows the individual stepping forward or will describe to me the image they see. Those who are not visual may feel their presence or simply know who is there. This is always an emotional moment. Tears quickly flow when an individual feels the intense love and begins to understand that they are not alone as they seek healing.

Along with recognizable loved ones, angels of light often come to assist. These beings are described in many ways and I believe they appear in the way that will most deeply resonate with the individual they are coming to serve. Often they are seen as hovering slightly above the ground, glowing with a brilliant white light, and wearing white robes. That being said, they've also shown up in other ways wearing a variety of clothing and colors. There is one common denominator between all sessions that I have witnessed; when a being of light shows up, only love and acceptance is felt. They never radiate judgment or illicit feelings of shame. They seem to have only one purpose: to help uncover and restore the beautiful light within, guiding each individual back to an understanding of who they are. They guide individuals back to Love.

Another common occurrence is for animals to appear in session. Many individuals have a deep love for their pets. The pets share this love and it creates a strong bond. The spirits of these animals often appear to assist in healing. This usually triggers even more tears than Grandma and Grandpa showing up! Animals radiate an energy of unconditional love. This powerful love can activate deep healing within a person's body and soul. I'm always glad when I see that surprised look on their face and hear them say, "It's my cat. Oh, it's my cat." And then I smile as the healing tears begin to flow.

There is so much going on beyond what we can see with our physical eyes. There are angels and loved ones working tirelessly to help us, guide us, and bring us the healing we seek. Heart-Centered Hypnotherapy sessions are a beautiful place to begin strengthening our connection with these loving sources and to claim the help and healing they are offering.

Larissa, age 53, has incredibly low self-esteem. She lacks self-confidence and is also very unhappy in her current life situation and relationship. She expresses that her marriage is lonely, and that she has never felt supported or truly loved by her husband.

Following these feelings, simply find yourself moving back to the source. Go back to one of the first times you felt these same or similar feelings. I'm not good enough. I'm a failure. I'm unsupported.

L: I'm 7. I just completed a gymnastics tournament. I performed so poorly *(the tears begin to brim)*. My mom's not here, only my coach. She's angry. She says, "Don't cry! Never let people see you cry. If you're going to cry, go where no one can see you." *(The tears stop but her voice is shaking)*

What are you feeling here?

L: So disappointed. I feel so sad. I'm embarrassed I did poorly and I'm embarrassed to cry. I feel sad that she's angry. *(Pause)* I feel unsupported.

Express this feeling of being unsupported. Speak out and talk to whoever it is you want support from.

L: I would like it from my coach, but *(pause, and choking on the words)* I really want it from my mom. *(Pause again and the tears are no longer held back)* Mom, I needed you there. I needed you to be there. I want to feel accepted by you. I don't feel loved by you. *(She immediately stops and holds her breath)*

What are you feeling now?

L: I hear her response, "That's silly. You're being silly. You don't need my acceptance or my love." I feel so alone. I am not supported. It feels so hopeless.

This feeling came even earlier than this experience. Keep moving back now, back to the source, an even earlier time when you made this conclusion that you're alone and unsupported.

L: I'm 2. I've just completed my first gymnastics lesson. My parents are both here. My mom tells me I did well. She says that someday I'll be great and she'll be proud of me. I feel happy she's paying attention to me. She doesn't very often. My dad even smiled at me and put his hand on my head.

This feels very positive. What conclusions did you make here?

L: Yes, I feel that right now they love me. *(Pauses and the tears gently flow)* But I also realized that their love is conditional. I decided that the only way to be accepted and loved is to do well in gymnastics. *(Pauses and cries another moment).* Love is always conditional.

I'd like to follow these emotions forward now. I'm inviting your Highest Self to guide you to another time or place that will help you understand how this early conclusion is still affecting your life.

L: I'm 17. I just lost the National Competition. I couldn't focus. I'm a failure. I don't want to compete anymore. I'm tired. I can't do this. I feel frustrated and angry toward myself. This was my chance and I blew it. I can't do it again. I'm just a failure. I'm too tired. *(Voice trails off into tears)*

When you made the decision to quit, that this is the end, what did you decide that means about you or your life?

L: I'll never have my parents' love. I'm not good enough. I will never be supported. I'm on my own. I am alone.

Can you see this affecting your current life and relationships?

L: It's the same in my marriage. I can't turn it around. I'm too tired. I'm on my own. His love is conditional. I'm not good enough. I can't do everything and be everything all the time. I'm failing.

Larissa, positive change in your current life will be possible as you learn to forgive and heal the past. This broken child part inside of you believes she is lovable only with condition and that she will never be enough and that is exactly the type of relationships and circumstances you are attracting into your life. It's understandable that you often feel alone, discouraged, and without value. Today, we can begin to change this. We can begin teaching this child part within you her true value.

(We walk through several self-forgiveness exercises to release the weight of discouragement and self-disgust. We invite white light to wash through her to fill the cracks and wounds that past experiences have created. I then invite her to welcome a loving source to come forward, to continue teaching and helping her to heal)

L: It's my Uncle Charles. *(She breathes deeply and shows a deep emotional connection to his presence)* He's been gone a long time. He was always so gentle and loving. We're standing on the top of a mountain. I see the water. It's calm. The air is crisp and cold but the sun is warm.

What message does your Uncle Charles have for you?

L: *(She is very quiet and then a look of relief washes over her)* He says I'm capable, that I'm always to remember that I am capable. He says it's my time to heal, that it's ok to let go of the pain of the past. I'm capable of creating a better present. He wants me to always stay in the present moment. I don't need to linger in the past or pine for the future; instead I can find peace by living in each moment and allowing myself to be guided in each step.

Is there a new affirmation you'd like to choose for your life? Any statements you want to claim as truth today?

L: I am capable. I am lovable and it is unconditional. I choose to let go and let God. I live in each moment and am guided by the Light.

Jyoti Ma

Harry, age 62, came into my office for help with weight release. He's been overweight since early in childhood. He has never been able to stick to a diet or exercise plan and is miserable when he tries to. As he's aging, he's beginning to experience the negative side effects of being overweight but is struggling to find the desire to alter his food intake.

Harry, I invite you to go to a recent time when you found yourself eating even though you weren't hungry. Without any effort, simply find yourself there and begin to sense and feel all that is going on around you.

H: I'm at work. I'm so bored. I'm concentrating on my work in my office, all alone. It's like the food from the vending machine is calling to me. I decide to buy a pack of cookies.

Focus on that feeling in your body. You said you were so bored. But you were working, so you couldn't have really been bored. I invite you to breathe into the feeling in your body and ask what the emotion truly is.

H: I'm lonely. *(His eyebrows go up in surprise and he says the words as though understanding their truth for the first time)*

Now find that feeling of being lonely in your body. It's there. Simply breathe into your body and that emotion of loneliness will present itself to you.

H: It's in my chest. It feels really tight. And heavy.

As you focus in on this feeling, I will help you find its source. Simply breathe into the emotion and allow yourself to easily be taken to

another time and place. I will continue to guide you, simply let me know when you get there. *(I watch as Harry's demeanor begins to change. The gruff exterior of this 62-year-old gentleman begins falling away, to be replaced by a tender, innocent, and younger essence)*

H: I'm 4. I'm at home and there's no one to be with. There's a yucky feeling in my chest. I want to relax, but I feel like I need to be on guard. I'm so tense. I don't know what's going to happen.

Harry, who do you want to be with you? Is there someone you need to call out to?

H: *(Nearly shouting, and with much emotion)* Mom! Don't leave me! Talk to me. I don't want to be alone! I don't want to be alone! *(He stops shouting and begins to cry)*

Did you make any conclusions here about yourself or about your life?

H: I'm going to be alone. I will eat to feel better. *(Again, his eyebrows go up and he's surprised by this insight)*

How is this decision still affecting your life?

H: I made food my only friend. I've never even had another friend. It's all I've had. Mom is gone so much. Dad has never been here. Food helps me feel better. I don't feel lonely when I eat. I guess I'm still using food to help me not be lonely.

Is this why it's been so difficult to change your eating habits and to lose weight?

H: I'm afraid if I stop eating treats, I'll feel lonely all the time.

Harry, I'm really proud of you for finding a way to cope with loneliness and difficult emotions. It helped you make it through a lot of tough times in your life. But, now, eating sweets to fill an emotional need is impacting your health and hurting you so it's time to choose a healthier way to address the loneliness. I don't have

the answer for you, but if you simply breathe and wait, someone will step forward to help you.

H: My grandfather is here! He died when I was very young. Why is he here?

Ask him.

H: Why are you here, Grandpa? *(Pause and a smile)* He loves me and wants to help me. How are you here? I missed you when you died. I've been so alone. *(Pause and then tears)* He says he has always been here with me, and that he watches over me.

I would like to thank your grandfather for being here with you and invite him to hold you. As he holds you, Harry, ask him to help you come up with three things you can do when you're lonely instead of turning to food.

H: *(There's a new light radiating from his face as he visualizes being held by his grandfather)* We've decided I need to always ask myself first if I'm really hungry or if I'm not really hungry. If I am, I should eat. If not, I can stand up and take a walk until the craving passes. I can reflect on my surroundings and be fully present in my life. And what he really wants me to do is to reach out to another person in some way. Maybe a kind note, a phone call, or a random act of goodwill.

Do you feel comfortable with these options? Are you willing to try out this new behavior for the next week until your next session?

H: Yes. I really think I can do it. It feels really good. It feels right to do this for myself.

Before we end, I invite your grandpa to help you choose a new guiding affirmation for your life. He may also share with you any words of wisdom he may want to offer you.

H: I am at peace. (*Deep breath, a sigh, and then a smile*) I wait before I react to anything. I think about the sea and the waves to reconnect me with peace and truth. I eat only when I am hungry and choose to connect with others in a healthy way rather than turning to food for comfort.

Chapter Six

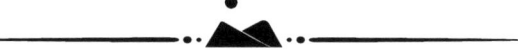

God's Role in Healing

"You are a divine being, directly connected to God."

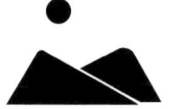

In conversation a few weeks ago, a client told me with surprise, "I never thought I'd find God by coming to therapy. But I have. It seems to be what it's all about; God's power is what brings the healing." I smiled as he realized this truth.

All healing occurs through a Higher Power. Although many titles are used to recognize this Higher Power, the most well-known title is God. Without God, there is no healing. It is impossible to have deep and lasting change in body and soul without God's power and grace. As a Heart-Centered Hypnotherapist, I am a facilitator of healing and a channel for light, but am not the Source.

What's really wonderful is that God's light and healing are available to each one of us, no matter where we are or what we've done. Our *understanding* of God does not determine our ability to receive His healing power. It is available to all who seek it with hope and humility. God loves each one of us unconditionally.

I have met with clients from a variety of backgrounds, religions, and spiritual understandings. I have visited with those who are deeply connected in a personal way to God and others who have a very loose idea of who or what God may be. And what continues to amaze me and bring me profound peace is that God finds a way to meet people exactly where they are and to touch them in a way they can understand and relate to—no matter the name they may know Him by.

When I am working with a client, I simply invite them to begin connecting with their Higher Power. I explain to them that this Higher Power is anything they believe in that is greater than them. There are many names used and even words, such as Love and Grace, to describe this Higher Power. Many individuals in a trance will immediately receive an image, a name, or a feeling to help them begin connecting with this Higher Power. Other times, the relationship develops very slowly and only with continual patience and effort. It always comes together in a way that serves the client's highest good. Whether they receive an image and name for God right away or whether it takes time, it's just right.

God knows you. And God loves you. I get to feel His love as it flows into sessions and it is amazing. God loves us enough to meet us where we are and then guides us by the hand in coming to understand the love and grace available to us. Our relationship with and understanding of God develops over time, as we continue to seek healing and positive change in our lives. As this relationship develops, it sparks a remembrance of our own inner light, divine potential, and infinite value. When we remember our value and feel divine love, our ability and willingness to welcome healing expands.

The following sessions will help illustrate what I am striving to describe. Each client is unique in their understanding of their Higher Power. The name we use does not matter nearly so much as does our heart and intention. God can lead us to where He is by meeting us right where we are.

Kate, age 30, came to therapy seeking to discover why she is so hard on herself. She demands perfection of herself and pushes herself to the point of exhaustion constantly. She has a deep-seated fear of making mistakes. She also has a severe addiction to sugar and feels that it is related to the emotional issues.

Kate had some resistance to the hypnosis induction. It took quite a bit of time to help her relax into an adequate hypnotic trance. She pulled in and out at times, jumping back to her conscious mind. With some time and patience she was able to access her earliest memories and we were able to get to the core issue.

K: I am lying in my crib. I'm only a few weeks old I think. I'm all alone and wearing a really pretty, white nightgown. My crib is white. I'm staring at the wall. *(There is a noticeable shift in energy. Kate begins to sob, completely overwhelmed with intense emotion)* I don't want to be alone. I feel so alone. I can't be here. Why do I have to be alone?

Kate, call out and tell your parents you need them; that you don't want to be there all alone.

K: Mom, where are you? Why aren't you here? I don't want to be alone. Dad! Come get me. Please, I'm so lonely. *(She suddenly stops and begins speaking to the hypnotherapist)* No, that's not it. It's not them. I'm not lonely for them.

Kate, allow yourself to drop into that emotion of loneliness. Be there in that moment and fully experience the emotions and explore where they are coming from.

K: It's God. I miss God. *(Sobbing from the depth of her soul now. Her entire body is shaking and tears are gushing from her eyes.)* I miss God. I miss Heaven. *(Voice shaking and words barely comprehensible)* I miss it so much. . . So much. . . I know I'm supposed to be here, but it's so hard. I don't want to be away from my Heavenly home.

How is this related to what you came here for today— the anxiety and need for perfection?

K: I have to make it back. I don't want to do anything that would stop me from getting back. I am so lonely here. I need to be sure I get back to Heaven.

Kate, this feeling is known as Celestial Homesickness. I want you to invite your Higher Power, God, to join you in your safe and relaxing place. I can't give you guidance to help you overcome this emotion, but He can. As I turn on this music you will feel His light and love washing over you. He will give you guidance and I want you to take note of the things He tells you so that you can share them with me when He's through. *(Nearly fifteen minutes go by before Kate speaks again, but it's apparent in her demeanor that she is having a spiritual experience)*

K: I'm OK now. I feel completely different.

Please share with me some of the important insights that you have been given.

K: God told me I'm doing a good job. *(She is choking back tears of joy and being overwhelmed with emotion; her words come a few at a time)* He told me it's OK to make mistakes, that it's why I am here. He told me that Jesus loves me and that, no matter what, as long as it's my true desire, I will be able to return to Heaven and be with them again.

Erin, age 62, came to hypnotherapy hoping to find more purpose in her life. She came with no belief in a Higher Power and has never received any religious or spiritual teaching. I invited her to simply open her heart and mind for her first session and to allow it to unfold without judgment.

Erin, find yourself moving to a safe and relaxing place. Find yourself somewhere beautiful and peaceful. Take all the time you'd like to be here, using all your senses to truly connect with this place. Once you're here, please describe for me what you see, sense, and feel.

E: I'm in a forest, sitting on a fallen tree. It's very quiet but I do hear sounds from small animals. Birds. Some squirrels. It's very peaceful. *(We spend several minutes connecting with this place and anchoring to the positive feelings found here before moving on)*

Now, I invite you to stand and walk down the path in front of you, beside the fallen tree. See this path and tell me how it appears to you.

E: It's like cobblestone. It's narrow but plenty large for one person to walk on. I see it winding down through the trees of the forest. There's a light up ahead, coming through the trees and touching down on the path.

Good. As you walk toward this light, you'll begin to see someone standing on the path. Take all the time you need and simply breathe your way through each step, drawing closer to the light on the path. Once you're there, describe for me what you see.

E: It's me, but younger. It's like how I looked when I was in my 30s.

This woman, me I guess, she looks really beautiful. She's radiating light and she looks really peaceful. She's got this gentle smile on her face and is looking right into my eyes.

Do you sense any qualities or characteristics radiating from her? Any positive feelings or emotions?

E: Yes. *(A small tear forms in her eye)* She is peaceful and gentle. She has this confidence but it's not overpowering. It's more like a gentle confidence. She's wise and loving. She isn't afraid and she isn't sad. She likes her life. She believes in herself. She knows where she wants to be and how to get there. *(Another tear drops from her eye)*

Erin, this is your Highest Self, the part of you that is eternal and wise. This is the part of you who sees clearly and strives to help you make good and healthy choices in your life. She is directly connected to your Higher Power. I'd like to invite you to continue walking down the path now. Allow your Highest Self to take you by the hand and to walk with you. I'd like her to guide you to your Higher Power. It will appear to you in a way that feels right, you simply need to walk down the path and see what comes.

E: *(She pauses for several minutes and then lets out a very deep sigh)* I see a mountain. When I came down the path, there was suddenly this large and beautiful mountain. The sun is reflecting off of it. No, somehow it's glowing independently of the sun. It's so bright and beautiful.

Beautiful. Notice any emotion radiating from the mountain.

E: *(Tears begin flowing and her voice trembles with emotion)* It's love. I've never felt love like this before. The mountain is glad I'm here. It's glad I came to see it. It's sending me so much love. I feel this love moving through every part of my body. *(She is sobbing tears of joy)*

Erin, this mountain is representative of your Higher Power. When you need strength and you desire to feel this love again, simply close your eyes and see this mountain. The energy of love radiating from

it is very real and very powerful. It is also unlimited. This mountain will work with your Highest Self to assist you in finding purpose and direction for your life. In time, your understanding of this Higher Power may expand and change but this is the perfect place to begin. Anchor now to this love by placing your hand on your heart. Breathe that love into every cell within you. And as you leave today, you will leave with pure, unconditional love helping to guide your life path.

Jane, age 43, feels isolated and alone. She expressed that she has many important people in her life, both family and friends, and yet she always feels like she doesn't belong.

What are you feeling right now?

J: I feel like I've been punched in the stomach. *(Her hands are cradling her abdomen)*

Give your stomach a voice and let it speak. There is no need to filter or hold anything back.

J: I didn't deserve that! You should've talked to me. I don't understand why. Why! I'm angry you didn't talk to me. You slammed me! You pretended. You're a liar and I can't trust you.

Follow these same emotions back to an earlier time with a similar experience.

J: I'm in middle school. Everyone is laughing at me. This group played a joke on me. It hurts so bad. *(She grabs her stomach again and her face shows that she's in intense physical pain)* Friends don't do this! I feel betrayed. I can't trust you anymore!

What conclusions did you make here?

J: I am unlikable. I don't trust people. They just pretend to be my friends. *(Pauses and then continues)* But I think these feelings came earlier. It's like this experience just reminded me I already knew these sad things about myself.

Then follow those feelings back again. Follow the sadness, betrayal,

and inability to trust back to the source. Gently allow yourself to be guided back. You're safe. It's a safe time to go back to the source.

J: I'm being placed for adoption. I'm not wanted. They're giving me away. *(She rolls onto her side, again clasping her stomach. The pain has increased)* I don't understand why! *(So much sadness and desperation in her voice)* I don't understand why you don't love me. It's not fair! Please! Please don't leave me!

And as you were taken away for adoption, what conclusions and decisions did you make?

J: I am not lovable. I have to be good. I have to follow the rules so I will be safe and no one else will abandon me. People will always pretend and their love will never be real. But if I'm good, I will be safe.

Jane. I feel like there's someone who may have something to tell you today. I invite you to simply breathe and return to your safe and relaxing place. Invite the peace, calm, and safety to surround you. Then tell me who joins you there. *(She is quiet for several minutes. Her pain begins to lessen; calm returns to her face. Then she begins to cry—large, full tears flowing from both eyes)*

J: It's God. He's here. I can't believe He's here. Oh, He's holding me. I can feel Him holding me. *(She continues to cry; the overwhelming feeling of love that God brings to her is apparent in her face)*

Jane, what does God want you to know?

J: *(Barely whispering)* He says I'm beautiful. He says I'm sweet and very lovable. *(She begins to smile)* He says... *(Pause, holding back a sob)* He says He loves me. He says it wasn't me. It was circumstances. *(Another pause)* He says they wanted to let me have a safe, stable, loving home. They didn't feel they had any other choice. But they love me and want what's best for me.

What's happening now, Jane?

J: He's placing His hand on my heart. He's restoring my innocence and ability to feel love. He's taking the black pain out of my stomach.

If these negative feelings try to return, these feelings of being unlovable and betrayed, what can you do to remember this love?

J: I can take a walk and reconnect with nature. I can soak in a hot tub and remember this warmth. I can let my husband hold me and ask to share God's love with him. I feel so happy right now. I feel so much peace. I can do this. I can keep this. *(Pause)* I am lovable. I deserve love.

Chapter Seven

Addiction From the Inside Out

*"If you desire to end an addiction,
seek to mend your soul."*

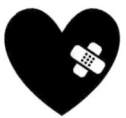

Many individuals come for hypnotherapy with hopes they can get help in healing from addiction. Addiction quickly darkens lives and blocks light. We can get lost in addiction before even realizing we have gone off course. Suddenly we look up and find ourselves wandering in a place far from where we ever intended to be.

Our addictions are coping skills. They are used to fill a void within us. Addictions are our substitute for true happiness and connection. The positive feelings they bring in the moment always come at a price. Sometimes this price is very great. Our health, financial security, relationships, self-respect and integrity are often in jeopardy when addictions take control.

Heart-Centered Hypnotherapy is highly effective with addiction because it strives not only to change the behavior but also to understand and heal the root cause. Our inner child has often chosen the addictive behavior because it believes it helps us in some way. The child has learned to mask pain, fear, discouragement, loss, self-loathing, and other negative emotions with the positive feeling and instant gratification the addiction brings.

A young child does not have the cognitive ability or wisdom to understand all the consequences of his behavior and our inner child is the same. The appeal of instant gratification is too great. A child will nearly always swipe a cookie from an open cookie jar. Our inner child will continue to choose the addiction until he is taught, *and understands*, why another choice is better.

The addictive substance or behavior may vary greatly, but the root cause is always the same. There is a fragmented young child inside the addict who is hurting and who found a way to help stop the pain. Those struggling with addiction are seeking connection and true happiness. The addiction, however, blocks both of these things from being possible. Until the inner child knows this, all the rational thinking and goal setting in the world will not stop the addiction.

Heart-Centered Hypnotherapy treats addiction by helping to find and heal the wounded inner child. The inner child must be on board with the decision to give up the addiction and try something new in order for true healing and lasting positive change to occur. This is why so many individuals try with so much valiant effort but continue to fail in releasing addiction for good. Addiction is not a conscious problem and so it cannot be solved with only the conscious mind. Instead, to really heal, one must be willing to dive deeply into the subconscious and heal from the inside out. Heart-Centered Hypnotherapy makes this possible.

Cory, age 60, has struggled with pornography addiction and low self-esteem throughout his life, despite coming from what he describes as a loving and stable family. He began sessions with the hope of understanding his behaviors and these long-standing negative feelings.

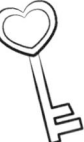

Focus now on the feeling of loneliness, the feeling of self-loathing. These two emotions continue to show up together. Without any effort, find yourself moving back, back to the source of these emotions within you.

C: *(With tears already brimming from his eyes)* I'm a baby.

Are you in the womb or outside of the womb?

C: *(Choking back sobs, he takes a few moments to respond)* I was just born. They are upset. My parents are upset. My mom is crying.

Cory, allow yourself to breathe. Be back in this experience fully and feel these feelings again.

C: I have a physical deformity. They're so upset. They are worried everyone will think I'm ugly.

(We take some time to continue processing and expressing his feelings and experience)

Cory, did you lose a part of yourself here? Was anything left behind?

C: Yes.

Breathe and look around until you find it. You'll know it when you see it.

C: I already see it. It's my ability to feel loved. It's my self-confidence.

When this part of you broke off, what did you accept in its place? What came to fill that void within you?

C: Self-loathing. I realized that I would never be as good as my brothers. I knew my parents would never love me. I feel so lonely.

You took on self-loathing and loneliness at this time, is this correct?

C: Yes. I wanted so badly to come here. But now that I'm here I feel so sad. I will always be lonely. No one can love me because I look this way.

Cory, who does this baby trust? Who can you call on to help this baby?

C: God.

Call out and ask God to help you take this baby somewhere safe and beautiful. Where does He want to take you?

C: He just wants to hold me.

OK, Cory, that's good. Let Him hold you.

(Suddenly he begins to cry. He's completely overcome with emotion and his entire body is shaking)

C: It's my mom. She's here too. She wants to hold me now. She wants me to know she loves me. She is so sad that her surprise and dismay at my physical deformity has hurt me so badly. She's telling me, "I always loved you. I was so tired in that moment. Please forgive me. Please let this go. Please know it's OK. You are beautiful. I love you."

C: God is holding both of us now. Me as a baby and my mom. He's helping us to heal.

By the end of the session, Cory was ready to reclaim the lost parts of himself. As he breathed back in self-love and acceptance, his entire countenance changed. He radiated peace and light—a 60-year-old man with the light and beauty of a pure and innocent infant.

Sam, age 37, came in for help with a gambling addiction that has created financial stress in his life. He has spent much of his adult life without consciously feeling any emotion. He says many have labeled him as "unfeeling".

Where are you?

S: It's last night. I'm driving by the casino and it's like I'm being drawn in. I don't feel like I have a choice. I have to go.

Find yourself in the emotion before this moment. What were you feeling before you saw the casino? Breathe, some part of you knows, even if you didn't consciously acknowledge it.

S: Discontent. Discontent with my position in life. There's also fear. And boredom.

Sit with these feelings for a moment. As you acknowledge them, notice which one seems to grow, seems to be at the core.

S: *(After a pause)* Fear. Fear I'm not enough. Fear I'm not doing good enough with my life. Fear that I'm just a loser.

That's what we're going to follow back now. Simply find yourself going back to another time and place.

S: I'm 8. I'm scared. I'm being punished for failing in school. *(He pauses and I encourage him to express the words and feelings he has directly to those within this experience)* Dad, I don't like it when you hit me. *(Holding back tears but his voice is shaking)* I don't want you to do that. I'm sorry for not living up to your standards. I'm afraid, Dad. I'm afraid of you hitting me. *(The tears break through)* I miss my mother. I miss Mom. I miss her so much. I'm so tired of being alone. I miss your attention. I'm sad that I'm alone. I'm trying, Dad. I'm trying but I can't do it.

What conclusions did you make here, Sam?

S: I want life to end because it would make the pain stop. Life hurts too much.

What decisions about your behavior did you make?

S: I decided to stop feeling. I can't kill myself because it's wrong. But I can stop feeling. I can lock up my feelings and not have to feel anymore. It hurts too much to feel.

What does this decision have to do with your addictive behaviors in your life?

S: They help me to block the bad feelings. When I'm involved in my addictions, it's like the pain goes away and I don't have to feel anything bad. My addictions protect me. Gambling. Food. Alcohol. They protect me from these feelings. I don't want to feel them. *(He pauses and then continues)* It's also how I punish myself for not being good enough.

In past sessions, we've begun to help you find the wise adult within you again. I'd like to invite him to come today. Is that alright? *(He nods)* **Find yourself leaving this painful experience and moving back somewhere safe, somewhere beautiful and calm.** *(His demeanor changes from one of sadness to one of peace as he moves into this new experience)*

S: I'm beside the ocean. The water is still and the sun is shining brightly. I see my Highest Self. He is smiling at me and welcoming me to come sit with him by the water.

I am going to give you some time to simply receive from him the messages he has for you today. When you are ready, please share with me what you learn. *(Several minutes go by as there is gentle music playing)*

S: Life can be filled with love. Choosing to block my emotions has also blocked me from positive emotions, emotions allowing me to feel connected to others and to feel love from them. Addictions hurt me. They block me from truth. They numb me and stop me from achieving the things I truly want to achieve. The mistakes of others are not my fault and I can forgive them and let go of the pain they cause. Love does make me vulnerable but love is still good. I've created this sad life I have by putting up walls so early in my life and shutting off my emotions. It's OK to feel again. As I choose to feel, I have power to create the life I want. I don't need to hide behind addictions anymore. I can choose a better path.

I'm very happy to hear these words. Does every part of you feel in agreement to this new path?

S: There seems to be some hesitation. Still some fear. But most of me wants this. Most of me wants to feel love and happiness again. Most of me now believes that life isn't just pain.

Would you be willing to put the fear away for just the next week, until your next session? For one week could you practice living your life without the fear and pain holding you back? For one week could you fully embrace this new way of living, trusting that you have power to create a happier and better life?

S: Yes. *(Big smile)* Yes. I can do that. I want to do that.

Your Highest Self is holding a box, do you see it? *(He nods)* **As he opens it, breathe all the fear and remaining pain into the box. He will hold it for you until you decide if you're ready to give it away for good.** *(He takes several deep breaths and then releases the energy of fear into the box)*

S: I am lovable. I am good. I have power to create the life I want. I am free.

Chapter Eight

Our Relationship with Food

"To truly transform your health and increase your vitality, fill your body with love."

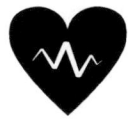

Food addictions are no different than any other addiction in many ways. Early in life most of us were taught to turn to food for emotional reasons. In nearly every culture, food is used for bonding and celebration. There is hot cocoa to warm the body and soul after playing in the snow with family and friends, cake to honor the birth of a loved one or co-worker, and countless other celebratory reasons to eat. From our earliest moments, food is used for connection and comfort. A child suckling his mother's breast finds comfort, love, and peace as he fills his tummy. As the child gets older there is ice cream after a heart break or cookies to compensate for a difficult day at school.

Having an emotional connection to food is understandable. It's impossible to avoid because we have to eat and it's such a huge part of life and culture. And it's not necessarily a bad thing. The trouble begins when we disconnect from the reality that food is simply a *part* of the bonding experience and instead attach to the false belief that *food itself* is our friend. Eventually, one often learns to skip the interpersonal connection altogether and go right to the food when feeling disconnected or out of balance.

This is when food addiction and unhealthy behaviors take root. We begin to rely on sweets, familiar foods, and beverages to make us feel better. When we're craving connection and feeling lonely, we turn to food instead of a loved one. When we're feeling sad or unworthy, we turn to food instead of asking for forgiveness or understanding. When we're feeling unsafe, we turn to food instead of reaching out to those around us to create a better environment. We learn this behavior at such a young age that we've developed the ability to self-medicate with food without even consciously acknowledging our reasons for doing so.

Eating for emotional reasons eventually catches up with us. Our weight, health, and vitality are affected by the types and amounts of food we eat. We begin to see negative effects appearing with our body and we begin to feel insecure. Over time, our relationship with our body becomes unhealthy and we see it as our opponent rather than our friend. We strive to conquer it with diets and exercise and we try to be the shape and size the media says we should be. We set goals and have every intention of eating better and giving up old behaviors of over indulging.

Simultaneously, we sabotage these goals because the inner child begins to panic. Food is their friend, remember? Food has become an important coping skill. We don't know how to give it up and subconsciously we don't even want to. The never ending battle within goes on and on. Weight comes and goes, emotions bounce up and down, self-confidence fluctuates with self-loathing, depression seeps in, and the willpower to deprive ourselves of what we want is the focus, rather than self-love.

Alternative beliefs and conclusions can also attach to food. Food, instead of being seen as a friend, may also be seen as the enemy. It can be seen as evil or bad. It can be seen as a way to punish ourselves when feelings of unworthiness go deep. Eating disorders such as Anorexia Nervosa and Bulimia are always attached to false conclusions about food as well as underlying false beliefs about the self. These disorders often stem back to trauma and abuse, or at minimum, negative beliefs about oneself drawn during early or painful moments and experiences.

Food addiction and emotional attachment to eating is not a simple issue. It's something that many of us struggle with. The more we come to understand our internal struggle and seek to heal the emotional wounds of our past, the easier it becomes to change unhealthy patterns and beliefs and to invite healthier behaviors to replace the old. Healing our relationship with food and with our body goes hand in hand with healing our soul. As we learn to truly love ourselves and see our body as our friend, our destructive eating habits shift in rapid and drastic ways. Heart-Centered Hypnotherapy helps accomplish this reality by looking deep within and healing from the inside out.

Seeing a Heart-Centered Hypnotherapist for private sessions is a wonderfully effective way to discover and heal subconscious reasons for retaining weight and clinging to unhealthy eating patterns. Also, the Trim-Life® program developed by Diane Zimberoff, is a powerful group class that uses Heart-Centered Hypnotherapy and focuses on achieving and maintaining a healthy weight. It is facilitated by specially trained providers. You may search for a private Heart-Centered Hypnotherapist or a Trim-Life® provider by visiting The Wellness Institute website: www.wellness-institute.org.

As in-person sessions are not an option for everyone, I've personally created several online classes to help with food, weight release, and body image issues. As a practitioner, my purpose is not to play into the idea that everyone needs a supermodel body and that zero percent body fat determines our worth. Instead, my purpose is to help people heal the false beliefs and unhealthy emotional attachments to food and also assist in developing a positive connection with the body.

My *21 Days to Love Your Body* online course, full of powerful guided meditations, is the ideal way to begin shifting your energetic vibration to one of greater health and vitality. Supplemental courses to help curb sugar cravings and subconsciously shrink the stomach are available as well. Perhaps my favorite class in this category is *Get Your Child Back on Track: Hypnosis for Healthy Eating*. With this course, parents can help their children learn how to tune into their own body signals in order to maintain a healthy weight throughout their life. You may visit my website to learn more: www.healingforlifewa.com.

As we heal the wounds of our soul and learn to listen to the needs of our body, we naturally make healthier choices with food and begin a positive shift toward greater physical and emotional health.

Trenton, age 27, began hypnotherapy with the intention of better understanding his anger and feelings of worthlessness. He also struggles to develop meaningful intimate relationships. He has been overweight since early childhood.

Where are you now Trenton?

T: I'm in a grove of trees. There's thick grass underneath and fluffy clouds above me. I feel so calm, just lying on my back. *(He is still and has a very gentle smile curving just the sides of his mouth upward. His breath is steady and calm)*

In this place we're going to begin getting in touch with your Highest Self, the wise adult within you. *(We take a few minutes to do this)* **Now that you've begun this connection, allow him to take you to another time and place, a time in your life where he was with you to help you make a healthy choice for your life.**

T: It's when I decided to stop smoking marijuana. It felt so good to walk away from it. *(He pauses and then moves into another time and place)* He also was with me when I decided to tell my mom that there was an older boy touching me. *(The calm turns to sadness. . .and then to anger)*

I feel that you're getting angry. Can you express these feelings please?

T: I tried to tell her about the abuse. She just cut me off, almost like she didn't hear. She didn't care. She changed the subject. *(He's yelling now, his anger very deep. I encourage him to speak directly to his mother)* Mom, I feel betrayed that you didn't take more action when I told you what was happening. *(Still yelling and hitting a heavy bag to help release some of the energy)* I feel so angry you wouldn't help me or talk about it! I feel even worse than before I told you! I'm angry that now I keep things inside and pretend that they're not valid or important. *(Pauses to catch his breath and the energy shifts. The anger is mostly released and a different energy washes through him)* I'm sad that you feel keeping up appearances is more important than helping me deal with this. It hurts so badly mom. I hurt so badly. *(And now the tears. With the anger released, the sadness and tears come in full force, washing down his cheeks like small rivers and choking on his sobs)*

Trenton, what conclusions did you make here?

T: I am not important. My emotions are less important than other people's.

And did you make decisions about your behavior or your life in this moment?

T: I won't share anymore. It doesn't help. I'll keep everything inside. *(Pauses and goes on, with a bit of surprise in his voice)* I also decided that eating more will make me big and strong. It will keep me safe- safe from being hurt. Food helps me feel better and it keeps me safe.

Trenton, is there anyone else you want to talk to? Other words and feelings you're holding inside about this experience? *(He begins to sob again and tells me he sees the bigger boy, the one who has been touching him)* **What do you want this boy to know?**

T: I'm so mad at you. *(His voice rises and the anger finds its way to the surface again)* I'm SO mad at you! You treated me like garbage! *(Yelling loudly and hitting the bag again as he continues)* You were never punished. I hate you for making me trust you. I hate you for abusing that trust. I hate you for getting away with it. *(And again, the energy shifts from anger to sadness. Tears flowing freely)* I wasn't good enough to protect myself. I wasn't strong enough to do anything to stop you. You made me feel so worthless and I am sad. I am so so sad.

(We spend the next thirty minutes visualizing washing this young

child part of him with pure beautiful water and inviting light into his being) **As you are being washed by this water and light, what are you choosing to release? What is being cleansed from your body and spirit?**

T: I'm releasing fear. I'm letting go of anger. I giving my hurt feelings to the Light. I am releasing sadness. I don't have to hold it anymore. I don't want to hold it anymore. It's time for me to heal.

Now notice who is coming to give you love and comfort today. What image or being is coming forward to be with you?

T: *(He begins to sob again, but this time tears of relief begin flowing from his eyes)* It's my grandfather. Oh how I love him. He died when I was little and I've missed him so much. *(I encourage him to be held and to listen to the counsel that comes)* He says I've been hiding and keeping things inside, trying to be what I think I ought to be, rather than who I am. He says to be open and honest- that it's time to talk about the things that hurt me and make me feel bad. He doesn't want me to keep these things inside. *(The tears increase)* He wants me to know that I matter, that I am important.

You released so much darkness and pain today. Is there anything ready to be restored? Or gifts ready to be received?

T: He's calling beautiful light from every direction. He says these are the parts of me that have been cleansed and are ready to come back.

Good. As he helps guide them back into you, please tell me what you're reclaiming.

T: I am reclaiming my playfulness *(Great big smile)*. I am reclaiming my ability to have fun. *(Pauses now and whispers)* I am reclaiming my willingness to be vulnerable, to trust. . . I am reclaiming my ability to be a kid, to play and have fun. *(Happy tears continue to stream and his countenance changes to peace and calm)* There is a column of light. It's the brightest light I can imagine. It's surrounding me. I'm being held inside this column of light. It's healing me *(Several deep sighs escape as this light finds its way through every part of him)*

Hold your hand on your heart now Trenton. Anchor yourself to this light. Breathe it deeply into every part of you. And when you're ready, I'd invite you to share with me your new conclusions and decisions about your life.

T: I am important. My thoughts and feelings matter. I am worthy of love and light. I can have intimate relationships. I can trust. I can turn to loved ones and friends to support and help strengthen me, rather than food. The Light will guide me.

Jesse, age 65, came in for help with food addiction. He finds himself constantly setting goals for healthier eating and then immediately sabotaging his goals. He is happily married but spends much time away on business travel.

We spent two sessions reconnecting with his Highest Self and also learning to tune into his body signals. The following excerpt is from his third session.

Jesse, where are you now?

J: I'm in the home where I grew up. I'm about five. I'm sitting at the kitchen table.

What can you see, sense or feel around you?

J: My mom is here. She's telling me to be a good boy and to finish my plate. It makes her so happy when I eat all my food. Dad just told me to eat another helping so I can be big and strong. My tummy hurts. I feel really full. But I don't want him to be disappointed.

What conclusions are you making about yourself here? Or about food?

J: We eat because it's time to eat. We always eat when it's time to eat no matter what. I need to eat because they want me to eat. My parents really want me to eat. It makes them so happy. I really like to make people happy. I feel happy when I make them happy so I keep eating even when my tummy is full.

I'm really glad you enjoy helping other people feel happy. That's very kind of you. But I'd like to invite your Highest Self to come and take

you on a little journey. Is that OK?

J: Yeah. That's OK.

Look across the room now. See who is coming in through the door. Do you recognize this person?

J: Yes, it's the same man I saw last week. The cool guy with big hands and a long beard.

I'd like him to take you on a journey. I invite him to show you what happens when you continue to eat to please other people and when you eat by the clock rather than when you're hungry, and when you keep eating after you're full.

(The man takes the boy by the hand and shows him himself as a teenager, overweight and embarrassed in gym class. He shows him in his early 20s, getting turned down by the army due to his poor physical condition. He shows him himself at his current age, unable to climb the stairs at work without getting out of breath and unable to play with his grandchildren because it's hard to stand on his feet very long)

Jesse, what are you learning by seeing these things?

J: I feel yucky and sluggish. I feel sad that my body feels so yucky. I don' feel happy.

You are a good boy and it was very kind of you to try to please your parents and make them happy by overeating all of the time. But now you can see that it doesn't make you feel good. You can see that it's hurting your body and stopping you from doing the things you want to do. Would your parents want that for you?

J: No, I don't think so. They said they want me to be healthy and strong.

What does your wise adult think? Does he have any advice for you right now?

J: He says I can eat when I'm hungry, that I don't have to keep eating so much. He says my body will feel better if I only eat when I'm hungry and not when I'm bored or trying to feel happy.

Does that sound OK to you?

J: Yeah I think so. I think I'd like to try it. I don't like what I saw and how yucky I felt.

Well then it's time to make a new conclusion about food. Something to help you make new choices with food and to help adjust your eating habits. You used to believe you needed to eat more than your stomach wanted in order to be happy and to make other people happy. You believed it was important to eat when the clock said it was time, instead of your body telling you it was time. What would you like to change these conclusions to now?

J: I am full. I am engaged in creating a healthy and positive life. I can choose when to eat and how much to eat, and I do so by listening to my body signals.

When you say these things, how do you feel?

I feel light. I feel happier already, like a real happy. I feel more energy too. My body seems excited to stop feeling so yucky.

Is there anything you'd like to ask your wise adult?

J: I would like to know if he'll help me learn how to eat better and to stop eating when I'm bored. . . He's laughing now. He says of course. We can do it together.

....

Stephanie, age 35, has struggled with an eating disorder since middle school. As soon as she thinks she's got it beat and her life headed in the direction she wants it, she finds herself compulsively bingeing and purging again. She feels completely helpless to stop the pattern, despite her conscious desire to overcome it and understanding of how it negatively effects her body.
....

(After some exploration and a few other regressions, she finds herself sitting on the floor of her living room listening to her parents talking in the kitchen)

S: My dad is telling mom she needs to lose weight. He's telling her she's unhealthy and looks like she doesn't care about taking care of herself. Mom is crying but agrees with him. She's really sad. She doesn't like her body.

(Without any prompting, Stephanie finds herself in another experience)

S: Dad's telling me I shouldn't have cut my hair. He says women should only have long hair. He says short hair is for boys. I already cut it. It's too late. I'm already ugly. He doesn't love me. He thinks I'm ugly. I'm fat and ugly. I'm not good enough. I won't ever be good enough.

(We move right into an energy release exercise, allowing her hurting and broken spirit fragments to say everything they've been holding back.)

S: Dad! Stop it! Stop it! I hate you! I hate that you make me feel worthless unless I'm skinny and have long hair! Don't you see you should just love me as I am? Can't you just accept me as I am? I'm your daughter! I feel worthless all of the time. I feel like I'm never good enough. I feel like everything is my fault and I will never please you. I hate that you've done this to me. This is all your fault. I'm so mad. I'm so mad I can't stand it. I'm so mad I just want to scream and hit and...

(Stephanie collapses and begins to cry. The anger and frustration are gone. Only sadness remains.)

S: Dad, I love you. Just please love me. Please just love me with short hair. Please don't make mom feel bad about her weight. She just wants you to love her. I just want you to love me.

Stephanie, thank you for allowing yourself to feel and express these things. I sense there's someone coming forward who wants to talk to you.

(A look of complete surprise washes over her face)

S: It's my dad. He's so sorry. He never wanted me to feel bad. He didn't realize his words were affecting me this way.

(She begins sobbing again but this time they are tears of relief)

S: He loves me. He's holding me. Oh my gosh, he's holding me and I can literally feel his love.

(We move through several other exercises including extending and receiving forgiveness. We also invite several broken spirit fragments to receive healing and then welcome them back into her core energy)

Chapter Nine

False Conclusions

"*Accepting a lie as truth is the foundation
of much pain within the soul.*"

We can't read minds. We also can't see into the depths of another individual's heart and soul. We can therefore never fully understand or empathize with why someone does the things they do or says the words they say. All we can do is interpret their words and actions based on our own perception, experience, and cognitive limitations. We often conclude another's words and actions to mean something about our self. We internalize these conclusions, making these beliefs a part of how we see our self and our life. In reality, our beliefs and perception vary greatly from the other person's thoughts or intentions. These misunderstandings carry a lot of weight. We call them false conclusions and they are the core of our pain— emotional, spiritual, and often even physical.

As an example, a woman in session the other day shared that she feels unimportant and unseen by her spouse. In trance she moved back to early childhood when her mother ran a daycare in their home. She found herself sitting on a rug in a room full of children where she was feeling sad and alone. She wanted her mother to hold her, to hold only her, but her mother was busy with another task. When her mother did come to hold her, she picked up two other children as well, placing all three of them in her lap for a story. This client, with her limited understanding as a child, concluded in this early moment: "I am just another one of the kids. I'm not important to my mother." This belief of being unimportant was still playing out in her current relationship.

I am not this woman's mother so I don't know what she felt or why she chose to run the daycare. But, I would bet money that this young child's conclusion was incorrect. This mother chose to run a daycare because her child *was* very important to her. It would be rational to believe that this mother wanted to be able to be with her daughter and actively involved in her life and development, but also needed a way to provide for her financially.

Our misperceptions and false beliefs cause us a lot of pain. They also help shape our expectations. Our expectations then help to create our reality. We attract into our life the things we are expecting and we see the things we expect to see. Our beliefs and misperceptions are the glasses we look through as we judge and strive to understand our world. Our reality is therefore very much affected by what we believe is truth. And what we believe as truth is often based upon a misperception or false belief. This destructive cycle is what we strive to put an end to with hypnotherapy- we seek to uncover these negative and false conclusions in order to heal the parts of us that believe them. We can then establish healthier beliefs and begin to walk our life path attracting the positive things we really desire.

Jason, age 52, feels discouraged. He expressed feeling that very little of what he does in his life actually brings him happiness, that he works 24 hours a day to please others.

Jason, where are you?

J: I'm four. Four was a hard year. I was lost at the shopping mall. I was so scared. I couldn't find my mom. And when I did find her *(Tears begin to flow and his voice drops to a whisper)* she was so angry. *(Pauses, as he moves fully into the experience)* She's blaming me. She is so mad and she's telling me it's my fault.

What do you want her to know? What words were you never given the opportunity to speak?

J: It's not my fault *(sobbing now)*. It's not my fault. You weren't watching me. Please, don't yell. Don't be mad. It's not fair. I didn't want to be lost. I'm scared, don't you see? Don't you care how I feel?

Did you draw any conclusions here?

J: I need to please her. What I feel doesn't matter.

I invite you to follow this conclusion, to witness another time and place that allowed this negative conclusion to truly take root.

J: It's later the same year; I'm still four. I have a little toy tractor and I love it so much. It's the best toy I've ever had. *(He stops and his emotions rise to the surface again. The tears start coming before he goes on)* We're at the airport. My uncle and his son came to pick us up. I'm with my dad. *(He pauses again, it's difficult to express because of how much pain he still feels)* My uncle's son wants my tractor. My dad makes me give it to him. He doesn't understand. It's mine. Dad says he'll get me another one but he doesn't know, this is the one that is mine. I'm throwing a fit. I'm so sad. Dad is angry and tells me I am selfish and I better shut up. *(Pauses)* And so I do. *(His tears suddenly stop and it's like a wall goes up, blocking all emotion)*

And what did you decide in this moment? What do you believe is true about you or your life?

J: That nothing is for me. I need to give everything away. I need to please other people. I have to give it all away. I can't have the things I want.

How is this still playing out in your life?

J: It's never changed. I still feel like I have to please others at the expense of myself. I give so much. I allow myself to be abused. I can't even defend myself. I'm so tired of living my life this way.

Would you like to change this conclusion? Would you like to claim something new for your life?

J: Yes, but I don't know how. It's just who I am, who I've been forever.

Not forever Jason. Inside of you is the eternal part of yourself, the part of you who sees clearly and who knows all you are capable of. This part of you knows who you have been and who you can choose to be. You've begun the process of connecting with this part of yourself in other sessions. Invite him to be here now, to teach you, this little boy, the truth about himself and his life.

J: He's here. He's strong and wise. It's crazy, he looks like me but really powerful and yet peaceful. He doesn't let others walk all over him. He stands up for himself and does the things that bring real happiness. He loves and cares for others, but doesn't allow himself to be abused by them.

Invite this wise part of yourself to teach you. What does he want you to know. As he speaks, tell me his words.

J: You are so handsome and smart. You are good. I love you just the way you are. You deserve everything that is good in this life. You are a good communicator. You can talk to all different kinds of people. You are intuitive and gentle. You can relate to others and their pain. You are unique. You are worthy of the greatest love, unconditional love. It's time to accept this love and to allow yourself to feel it within yourself. All that you need is within you. Look into your heart and find this beauty and goodness. That is where I am. I am here for you. You are me. And I am you. Everything you see within me, is already within yourself.

(I played some music as he continued to receive counsel and healing)
And now, Jason, what would you like to claim as truth in your life?

J: I am strong. I embrace and find my inner strength. I create my own happiness and I do so with love and joy. I can love and help others while maintaining my own self worth and integrity.

Rachelle, age 19, came in unsure of what she wanted to work on so we simply let her body and spirit guide her.

What are you feeling in your body now?

R: I feel a really tight knot in my stomach. It feels like it goes all the way through me.

Breathe into it and identify the emotion or feeling within that knot.

R: It's hungry. It's sad. It's confused and alone.

Rachelle we're going to follow these feelings back to the source. *(I begin counting her back and she quickly finds herself in another time and place)*

R: I'm so little. I think I'm 5 months old. I'm crying and crying. I'm really upset. My mom is upset. She's yelling at me. She's shouting "All you do is cry! Just shut up! Shut your mouth!" She's not trying to help me. I keep crying and crying. *(Her tears begin to flow as she feels the same emotions she had as a baby in this moment)*

What did you want your mom to know? What words and feelings are still locked inside you from this time in your life? Speak directly to your mother.

R: I just need your help. I'm really hungry. I'm hungry all the time. I'm not getting enough food to eat. I just want to eat. I feel so confused. And sad. I just want my hunger fed. I just want to eat. I'm so sad that you're not hearing me. I'm sad you're mad at me and don't want to be around me. *(Her tears continue flowing steadily)*

What conclusions did you draw here Rachelle?

R: I am always going to be hungry so I embrace the feeling of lack. I am undeserving of having my needs met. My needs cause others anger and frustration and so I will always choose to ignore my needs.

There may be a piece of you still here. Please look around the room and see if you can identify anything that represents a part of you.

R: I see a little girl hiding under the crib. She came from inside me. She doesn't want others to see her. She doesn't want them to know she even exists. She's so sad that she made her mom upset. She's sad that no one wants to help her.

Rachelle, this little girl is sad and afraid. She needs help. She needs to know she is important and safe. I invite you to become the nurturing and loving parent for this little girl, to give to her all that she's been needing and wanting to hear. Search deep within yourself and call on the nurturing and loving wisdom within yourself. When you feel ready, take this little girl by the hand and look her in the eyes as you speak. Be gentle.

R: I know you're sad and have been hurt. You don't need to be hungry anymore. There is always an abundance. No one will turn you away or judge you for asking for your needs to be met. Your mother was very tired. She loves you. She didn't understand and didn't mean to hurt your feelings. If you will come out of hiding now, others will help you and praise you and love you. It's time to smile again. I see you. I love you. Will you come with me? *(She tells me that the little girl is willing to come out of hiding)*

Guide this little girl back to your safe and relaxing place. Invite her to look up at the sky and to receive the healing light of the sun. Then please tell me what happens.

R: The light is washing through her. It's cleansing all the shadows and pain within her. *(She's smiling so big now. There is relief and joy apparent in her face)* She is so beautiful and clean.

If it feels like the right time, I invite you to ask her to come back, to join you again.

R: *(She reaches out to take the little girl by the hands and invites her back)* I am reclaiming the wholeness that I haven't felt in a long time. I accept feelings of abundance. I trust again in my truth. I am worthy of having needs and I am willing to express my needs.

How is having this part of you back going to affect your current life and relationships?

My boyfriend will be so happy. He'll be glad that I will be able to express to him my wants and desires. It will feel good to have an opinion and to honor my needs. I can be real again. I don't have to pretend. I am happy being me and can trust others to know my needs. I feel so good. I feel so whole.

Alesha, age 56, came in for a session after an argument with her husband. He had cleaned out a room in their home and thrown away several boxes without her knowledge. She expressed to me "My reaction was over the top. It was like I turned into a beast and I was violently upset. Nothing in the boxes was even important but I still feel very angry and sad. I don't understand why."

A: I'm at school. I think I'm in second grade. Everyone is talking about Christmas. They got many things.

And what are you feeling?

A: I feel confused. And sad. I didn't get any presents this year. I heard one girl say to another "I know my dad really loves me. He bought me the doll I really wanted." Everyone seems so happy. Their families seem to love each other. Maybe if we had more things, my family would love each other too. My parents fight all the time. I don't think they love each other. I don't know if the love me either.

What are you deciding about yourself or about your life here?

A: I want to have things. I can't throw anything away. The more things I have, the more love my family will have.

This part of you, the one that decided that things are important, is this who got so mad at your husband today?

A: Yes. She's worried he'll stop loving her. It's not good to throw things away.

I'm going to invite you to see this child part of you. Invite this little girl to come out of hiding so we can talk with her. Is she willing to

do so?

A: Yes. She's here. She's so young. And pretty. But sad and kind of looks dark.

Now, this little girl doesn't know me and probably doesn't trust me very much. And that's ok. But I'd like to invite her to look around and to see who is coming to help her. There is someone she trusts coming forward.

A: *(With tears and a voice of surprise)* There's a beautiful woman. An angel.

Beautiful. Is the little girl willing to listen to this angel? Does she trust her?

A: Yes. Very much.

I'd like to invite this angel to teach you and help you. Have her hold the little girl and tell me the words that come.

A: *(Repeating the words of the angel, spoken to the child)* You are very smart. I'm glad you found a way to feel love, even when it was so difficult. Collecting things and having lots of things has helped you to feel safe for a long time. And now there are better ways to feel safe, and loved. You decided that having things would help your family love one another, but now you can know a secret. Love has nothing to do with things. Real love is in here *(the angel puts the little girl's hand on her heart and covers it with her own)*. Real love is felt. Real love is beautiful and independent of any stuff. Having things has helped you survive and cope with tough feelings, but now you're old enough to know the truth. Real love comes independent of anything tangible. Your husband loves you. Your children love you. And they love you for who you are, not what you have. Your parents did the best they knew how. They struggle with a lot of darkness and pain, but I want you to know that deep within them is a light that shines bright and inside of that light is a beautiful love for you. Today, I bless you to release the pain and darkness of the past and to welcome light into your own beautiful heart. Would you like to do that? *(She nods her head)*

(As music plays, tears stream down her cheeks. She breathes in gently but deeply; with every breath she welcomes true understanding of love and releases her old beliefs about love being attached to physical possessions)

What new truth would you like to claim today?

A: I am lovable and I am full of love for others. I feel it in my heart and soul. I choose to feel this love now and always.

Chapter Ten

Looking Within

"When we are triggered by the behavior of others, it is a signal we have something within us longing to be healed."

Last night I sat in our family room with a friend who came to visit. She discussed a situation that has caused her a lot of stress. She is a member of a social group but has struggled to have a positive relationship with a particular member. Being in the same room with this individual feels stressful to her and she is resentful that this has stopped her from really enjoying the group.

I tried hard to restrain myself, but my inner therapist got the better of me and couldn't pass up an opportunity to guide her in a bit of self-reflection so I moved forward with her permission. Before I knew it, she was dripping tears and deep in a trance.

I used a relatively simple process called an emotional clearing. I had her speak to this other woman as if she were there and tell her the behavior that triggered her negative feelings and then we honed in on the emotion that came up inside of her chest. She identified it as feeling inferior. Under the obvious anger and resentment was a child part of her hurting and afraid that she wasn't good enough. This other woman's behavior triggered a deep negative belief in my friend that she is inferior. As we followed the feeling and belief back, she uncovered early experiences with her grandmother that led to this false conclusion about herself.

Emotional clearings help us gain clarity. When someone in our life triggers us in an emotional way, rubs us wrong, or causes a stir of something painful within us, we can be grateful to them. They are presenting us with the opportunity to look inside, to find and then heal the part of us that is wounded and hurting. If a boss, a co-worker, a friend, a spouse, a child, or a stranger can trigger a negative response within us, we have healing work to do.

What's amazing is that by doing the clearing and finding the deeper root of the issue, we can easily clear the energy with the current person in our life. Once we find and recognize the broken part of our self that is being triggered, their words, presence, or behavior simply stops having the same negative effect on us. When we are triggered emotionally, it says much more about us than it does about the other individual. We can use this realization to begin healing current relationships as well as our inner child.

Jaren, age 43, started coming to sessions desiring help with his temper. He has a son who is about ten years old whom he often feels frustrated and angry with.

Find yourself in a recent experience where you were feeling something negative. Simply breathe and allow your breath to guide you back.

J: It's yesterday. My son responded rudely and I flipped out. I yelled at him and sent him to his room. My stomach is in knots. I hate this. I hate fighting with him. I hate being angry.

Breathe into the knots. What would these knots like to say? What do they want your son to know?

J: I'm worried. I feel frustrated. I feel disappointed and angry at you. And at myself. I'm also afraid. . . *(He pauses and breathes in this realization)* I'm afraid. I'm afraid that people will see you as a brat. They won't see the good person you are.

Jaren, this is a feeling and belief that we want to follow back now. They won't see the good person I am. They don't see the good person I am. Breathe and allow yourself to be taken back to the source of this fear, this belief.

J: I'm five. Dad's angry that I wasn't listening. He's grabbing my arm and twists. It's hurting my wrist. I'm afraid. I'm afraid of the physical pain and punishment. He's taking me to my room and tells me to stay there. He is so mad.

Name some of your feelings and thoughts as you're here in your bedroom.

I'm scared. I feel bad about myself. I'm messing up. I can't do anything right. He doesn't love me like he loves my brother. He doesn't like to spend time with me. I'm bad. I am naughty. *(His energy shifts from sadness to anger)* The world is not fair. I am wronged.

What happened just now. Your feelings have shifted.

J: I see a rhododendron flower. It's wilted. It was my optimism, it's gone. There's a new energy, something heavy that's entered my body.

Allow yourself a moment to feel this new energy. Effortlessly you'll be able to identify its significance.

J: It's anger. When my optimism left, it made room for anger. Anger allows me to justify. It says it's not me, it's them. I am wronged. They are the problem.

And you've kept this anger with you since then. Is that correct?

J: Yes. It's easier to feel angry. It helps me be safe and feel better about myself. I just want to be accepted.

Jaren, I'm glad you found a way to cope with your sad feelings. And I honor you for doing the best that you knew how. Now though, I'd like to invite your Highest Self to come and teach you. Find yourself back in your beautiful place. Your Highest Self is there waiting for you.

J: Yeah, I see him. He's telling me that anger is all that the people see. It blocks them from seeing the real me. They can't accept me because they don't know me. He says it's not good for me to keep it any longer.

How do you feel about what he's saying?

J: I think he's right. But I don't know what to do about it. I don't know how to let it go. I've had it with me for so long and it has helped me.

Ask him for more wisdom.

J: *(Speaking very slowly and pausing often)* He says forgiveness is the answer, not anger. He says forgiveness protects me because it connects me with those I love. Anger separates me from them. Forgiving myself allows me to be innocent again. Forgiving others allows me to not judge or be judged.

(After several forgiveness exercises, Jaren has released enough of his anger to receive the following truths directly from the Light)

J: I am smart. I am loving. I am funny and caring. I love to help others. I choose to heal, to let go of selfishness and fear. I am not supposed to be in the dark anymore.

Where are you supposed to be?

J: In the Light. *(A beautiful smile spreads across his face)* I am meant to be in the Light. I am love.

How will this change or affect the relationship with your son.

J: I am meant to love him, that's all. I can teach him by loving him. I can allow him to make mistakes and love him. I can watch him grow and love him. I can let him be imperfect and love him. I can just love him. That's my purpose. That's my role. My anger stemmed from fear and my old beliefs that I am wronged. I choose to release these lies and to simply embrace love. Love and forgiveness. I AM LOVE! *(New tears come, but these tears are brought by joy)*

Patti, age 41, is a single mom of an 11 year old girl. We had met for a few sessions prior to this one. She wanted to focus on releasing anger and resentment toward her daughter.

Go to the recent experience with your daughter. Tell her what feelings you are feeling when she speaks and behaves in certain ways.

P: When you don't pick up your clothing, I feel completely disregarded. When you ignore me or don't do the things we have talked about, I feel resentful and like you don't care about keeping our environment healthy and clean. I feel angry that I'm not important to you. I feel angry that I care more about our relationship than you do. I hate it when you talk about how wonderful Julie's mom is and go on and on about her but then tell me I should just not talk. I feel so angry at you.

Now, breathe into the feelings of anger and resentment. Where in your body are you feeling these emotions? *(She holds her hands on her chest)* **Good. Now breathe into the feeling there and describe it for me.**

P: It's actually sadness. *(Her cheeks begin to flush and her eyes squeeze tightly)* I just feel sadness. I think the anger was a cover because the sadness is so painful. *(The tears flow gently down one cheek)*

Honor that feeling within you by giving it a voice. Allow that dark energy in your chest to speak the words and feelings it is holding.

P: I'm sad that I don't feel like I'm enough. I'm sad that I don't think I'm a good enough mom. I'm sad that she doesn't love me as much as I love her. I'm sad that we're losing our connection. *(By now she is openly crying and tears are streaming down both cheeks. She is very connected to the emotion of sadness)*

I'm going to help guide you back to the source of these feelings now. Simply allow another time or place to come into your mind as I do so. *(I help her regress, taking our time and honoring her painful feelings)*

P: I'm by myself in my house. I'm scared and sad and alone. I'm sad because nobody cares about me and thinks I don't matter. I'm sad because they are right- I don't matter. (deep sobbing)

Patti, we're going to keep going back now. I invite you to easily move back to the moment you make that conclusion, where you took on this belief that you don't matter. *(I continue to help her regress)*

P: I only see darkness. There's nothing around me but darkness. *(Long pause)* And I feel like I'm floating.

Be patient and allow yourself time to be in this darkness and feel the floating. If you listen, you may hear a sound. Please tell me when you do.

P: *(with total surprise and some excitement)* I hear a heartbeat. I hear my mother's heartbeat. Oh wow. I am so tiny. I'm just floating here listening to her heartbeat. *(The surprise quickly switches back to tears)* My mom is scared and sad. I think it's my fault. I'm the one that's bringing her these emotions. I don't know if she wants me. I feel like she really dislikes me.

What would you like to tell your mom? What would you want her to know?

P: If you could give me a chance, I would bring you a lot of joy. *(Her voice shakes and tears continue to fall)* I sense that she's not ever going to fully love me. It's not because of me, it's because of her. There's a block between us.

What do you believe is true about you?

P: I am worthy of love! I know I am. The world is confusing. People can't see me for who I am. I have to put a show on for people so they can attach to the outside of me. Letting them attach to the inside of

Jyoti Ma

me is too scary. It's OK if they don't like the outside of me because it's not the real me. But if I let them attach to the inside and they leave me, it'll rip me apart.

Patti, did you leave any part of yourself behind in the womb? Did you leave anything here for safekeeping?

P: *(With incredibly deep emotion and sorrow)* Yes. I left the core of my essence here. I can see it. It's a shining light of yellow, orange, and red.

As you look into this beautiful light, what do you know is true about yourself?

P: I have so much love. Oh, I have SO MUCH LOVE. *(She speaks with awe in her voice as she recognizes the depth of her core)* I am beautiful and powerful. I have a gift to empathize and understand others. But the black wall I've built around this core stops me from connecting. I don't truly connect with people- there's always the fear of rejection.

Patti, it's not the right time to fully reconnect with your core. Every part of you must feel safe before we can do so. But for today I would like to try to help this baby begin to heal. Please notice what person or being is stepping forward to help this baby today.

P: *(Again with surprise)* It's me. It's me but I look full of light.

Perfect. Please allow this beautiful part of yourself to reach out and hold this baby. Please look deep within yourself and find the love and wisdom this baby so desperately needs.

P: I see you. I know you are hurting. You are gonna be just fine. Things are going to come to you when you need them. You're never alone. Even you are not feeling loved, it's not truth. I always love you and I am with you. *(She pauses and again addresses me)* The baby is surprised. She's not sure what to think. She didn't know there was love available to her.

This is a brand new experience for this child and we are going to take it very slowly. Today, simply hold her and speak to her gently,

reminding her of the truth of who she is and that she is safe now.

P: Little one, the Universe loves you too. You have a purpose and it's not a mistake that you're here. You have wisdom within you that you have yet to tap into. *(She pauses again and addresses me)* There's a feeling of confusion. There's another voice telling the baby that this isn't real, that's it's a lie, and not to listen.

Patti, there's no right or wrong answer, but only your Highest Self may answer this next question. Does this voice belong to some part of you or to an energy outside of you?

P: No, it's outside of me. It doesn't belong to me. It's a yucky feeling. It's very dark. It's angry you're here.

(We spent the next several minutes working with this outside energy source and helping to separate it from the baby. Both the energy and the baby were hesitant to let go and afraid of being alone. In the end, with the help of the Light, the attachment left and the baby was blessed with the energy of dancing, music, and light to fill the void created by the outside attachment)

Patti, for the next two weeks I would invite you and this baby to try on a new and healthier conclusion. I would like your Highest Self to help you create a statement that she knows is true and you get to try it out until our next session to see how it feels and how it changes your life for the better.

P: I am worthy of being heard, seen, felt, adored, and loved. *(A large sigh)* That feels really good. I am worthy of being heard, seen, felt, adored, and loved. I like this. We're willing to accept it for two weeks.

Beautiful. I'm so glad. Claim it at every moment of each day and you will begin to feel a difference in your life. I also invite the Light to bless you with a filter over your eyes, so that each time you look at yourself in the mirror, you will see yourself through the eyes and love of God. In two weeks we will meet again.

It took several more sessions before Patti was healed enough to welcome back her core essence. When they reconnected it was a beautiful and amazing experience. The light could literally be seen radiating from her as she walked out of my office, fully embracing the truth of her value and worth, no longer afraid of connecting and being loved by others.

Chapter Eleven

Womb and Early Life Experiences

*"Be gentle with your little ones.
Every word, every thought, every experience
makes a difference."*

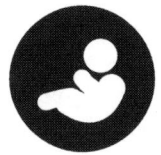

My first Heart-Centered Hypnotherapy training was a six-day intensive course where a group of us listened, learned, and then jumped right into some hands-on clinical experience using one another for practice. I'll never forget the first session I facilitated. Within seconds of going into a trance, my classmate was suddenly curled up in the fetal position and crying out that he was scared and it was so dark. I glanced at one of the supervising teachers with a questioning look and she said, "He's in the womb." My mouth literally dropped open. When I finally picked my jaw up off the floor I whispered to her: "Seriously? I didn't know that was even possible!" She smiled and helped me continue guiding the session.

Visiting very early experiences and moving back into the womb are both pretty common occurrences during healing sessions. These earliest of experiences can play a large role in our development and influence the way we see ourselves and the world around us. It's true that an infant has no ability to verbally communicate, nor does it posses the cognitive ability to process words and conversation. But the subconscious parts of them, including the energy and spirit, are aware and collecting information constantly. This information is gathered throughout life and stored within us. Infants and young children are extremely sensitive to the emotions and feelings around them and because their experience and understanding are so limited, they internalize everything as being about them. Negative conclusions and false beliefs are often accepted as truth.

As we recognize this unfortunate reality, we can take personal responsibility to heal from the misunderstandings of the past. Heart-Centered Hypnotherapy sessions help with this process. But, even on our own, we can challenge nagging thoughts and self-doubts whispered from dark corners within our mind, and begin to replace them with love and truth.

The following session excerpts will help you begin to see how vital it is that we are gentle with our tender children. You will also begin to feel the broken and hurting child parts stirring within yourself. Moving back to reflect on these earliest roots of pain and misunderstanding can lead to beautiful and deep healing.

Larissa, age 63, came to her session hoping to relieve feelings of loss and anxiety. She also expressed an inability to appreciate or even acknowledge her feminine side and has always found herself to favor masculine traits.

Larissa, do you have a spiritual connection. And if so, what do you call it?

L: Yes. Spirit.

Let an image come to you which signifies your highest or adult self within you.

L: I'm ageless. I am a big white horse.

Good. I want you to allow yourself to fully connect with this Highest Self and allow her and Spirit to be with you for guidance and protection during this session. Now, go to the most recent time you felt this anxiety and loss that you spoke of. Focus on those intense feelings; allow them to fully rise to the surface as you drop into this recent experience.

L: Jake died. Jake is my horse, my best friend and protector. I'm dreaming it but it's so real. He's getting old and will soon leave me. In my dream he is running and then just falls to the earth, leaving me devastated and alone.

Focus on being devastated. Alone. No one there to protect you. Allow yourself to go to one of the first times you experienced these emotions and fears.

L: I'm six years old. I'm standing in a wheat field by myself. I think

I'm dreaming this too. But it's real at the same time. In my dream the white horse picks me up and puts me on his back. He is meant to be with me, because I have no one else.

Let's focus on "having no one else". Pull up that emotion. What are the core feelings there. Where are you feeling it in your body?

L: Sorrow. Fear. Sadness. In my heart. My chest is swelling and so painful. *(Tears are coming up quickly and her breathing has become heavy and irregular)*

Sorrow. Fear. Sadness. Go to the source of these emotions. Find the first time you experienced them with this level of intensity.

L: I'm very little. I see only darkness. I'm not sure what's going on.

Give yourself a moment to be there. Ground yourself to this experience. Call on Spirit to help you be there and to understand what is happening.

L: Mom's too tired. . . It's too late. . . I'm already formed. I shouldn't have come but it's too late. I'm already here. I'm already inside of you!

Larissa, drop into the emotions of this experience and give that tiny baby a voice. She couldn't be heard inside the womb but we can hear her now and want to know what she has to say.

L: I've been set up. Coming into this life was going to be a benefit. My mom's too tired. She never says it; but I feel it. She's too tired and doesn't want me.

What early conclusion did you draw about yourself here and decision about your behavior?

L: I'm a bad thing. I'm selfish. I need too much. (Long pause) If I take care of myself, it won't draw too much. I don't want to be a burden. Everything I do is a burden. No one is strong enough to hold me.

(By the end of the session Larissa was able to release large amounts of negative energy and consequently able to form new and healthier

decisions and conclusion to begin affirming in her life.)

L: I came from a place of feeling and feeling is OK. The horses have been sent by Spirit to protect me and help me. Being masculine was my cocoon; a barrier that I placed around myself. But the essence inside me is beautiful and feminine and ready to be released. I am connected to my Big White Horse whether he is physically with me or not. Even when he dies, his spirit will be with me still as it was when I was a child. I am safe, protected and loved.

TRENT, age 40, is a husband and father of two young girls. He works in a high pressure job where he feels undervalued and unappreciated. He came to his first session seeking help for underlying feelings of anxiety and sadness. He has struggled with these feelings all of his life and desired to understand why.

He slipped into hypnosis quite readily and we were able to make some important discoveries.

Hypnotherapist - Go to a recent time you felt anxious; where you experienced this sadness and anxiety intensely.

Trent (T): I'm in my home. A file was corrupted that I needed for work. My daughter is sad. I am sad. I promised to spend time with her. *(Deep breath)* I have to redo this file. This is such a waste. There's not enough time. My daughter is crying. I'm breaking my promise. *(Speaking quickly, with anxiety and sorrow)* There's never enough time. I want her to feel worthy and loved. I'm making a mistake.

Where are you feeling this emotion, this sadness and anxiety?

T: In my heart, and here *(He touches near his pelvis, indicating the root chakra)*. There's something wrong with me; I feel pain *(he's now holding his stomach)*.

Travel back to the source of these emotions. Take yourself to the first time you experienced this sadness, this feeling of anxiety, this fear of not having enough time.

T: It's dark. It's tight. There's a bowling ball sitting on my stomach. . . No. . .it's poison. It's poison coming through my cord. It's heavy.

I don't understand. I'm afraid. *(Trent has regressed to his mother's womb and has balled himself into the fetal position)*

Listen and tell me what you hear.

T: *(Whispering)* I hear my mother's heartbeat. . . I hear the doctor telling her they need to stop the labor. *(Voice rising and getting more rushed)* I want to come out! I need to come out. My mom needs to know I'm a wonderful ball of light and I'm going to be just fine. She lost my brother before she was pregnant with me. I feel her anxiety and sadness for me, worried I won't be ok. She's been feeling so anxious and sad this whole time I've been growing. I want to come out and let her know I'm beautiful. . . But they're poisoning me. I can't get out. I feel myself dying. *(Screaming now)* Let me out! You're poisoning me! I don't have enough time! I need to come out now! I'm dying! I'm dying! Let me out! Please, please *(words drop off into heavy sobbing)*.

(We were later able to verify that due to early labor, the doctors had administered an alcohol based medication to which the baby had an allergic reaction to and did in fact nearly die.)

(After energy release and some processing, Trent is ready to be reborn, to create a better birth experience. He is curled up in the fetal position, face down, with my hands pressing against his head to imitate pressure from the birth canal. He wriggles and twists and pushes until he is completely stretched out. He rolls from his belly to his back, with head resting in my lap. With my hands gently cradling his head I whisper) **You made it. You are safe and loved and welcome. You are right on time. I love you.** *(Peace and joy wash over his face, the innocent demeanor of a child still present)*

T: *(After a beautiful healing exercise he chooses his new life decision and pattern)* I am awesome. I am a child of God. I create my own safety anytime I want. I honor commitments first to my children, to myself, and my wife. There is an abundance of time for the things I choose to do.

Rachel, age 46, began hypnotherapy with hope it would help her overcome depression. She came for several sessions before uncovering the deepest root of the problem.

Rachel, where are you?

(Before I even finish counting her back for an age regression, she is sobbing and shaking. Her entire body is shaking so hard it could easily have been mistaken for a seizure)

R: No! No! Noooooooooo! *(She is screaming at the top of her lungs. Her entire soul screaming every sound)* NO!!!!!!

Rachel, where are you?

R: I'm so sorry! *(The tears are flowing freely. Words barely escape between gasps and sobs. The shaking continues)* Please forgive me. I'm so sorry. I didn't know what else to do. I didn't know what else to do. *(The agony in her voice is indescribable. She is in incredible pain)*

(She begins rolling from side to side. Inconsolable. So many tears)

Rachel, how old are you here?

R: I'm 16 *(choking on the words, she continues)* I just had an abortion. I killed my baby! *(screaming again)* I killed my baby! They killed my baby and I let them. I felt it die. I don't know what to do.

Rachel, breathe into your body and find the emotions you are feeling. Tell me these emotions.

R:*(Her voice so weak, so hopeless)* I feel so much sorrow. I feel anger- at myself and at them. At my parents, at Bob, at the doctors, at my friends. . . *(and then she begins to sob again)* I feel guilt. I feel so much guilt. How could I let this happen. . . *(trailing off as her crying continues)*

Rachel, is there anywhere else your Highest Self wants to take you today? Anywhere else we need to visit in order to really understand all that you're feeling and need to release?

R: Yes

Find yourself easily and effortlessly going to this place. Breathe gently and find yourself moving back now, back to another time, another place to help you understand the guilt and depression and sorrow you've been feeling.

R: I can hear my mother. She's talking to my grandfather.

Where are you? How old are you here?

R: I don't know. It's dark. I feel very small. *(After a few moments she realizes where she is)* I'm in the womb.

Listen again. Tell me what you're hearing.

R: My mother is crying. My grandfather is screaming at her. He's so mad. He's really, really angry.

Tell me the words you hear.

R: "How could you do this? How could you go and get yourself pregnant? Of all the stupid things you could have done, why did you do this?" My mother is sobbing. She's so sad. I can literally feel her sadness. And her fear. It's overwhelming me. *(She stops to breathe, to calm herself enough to continue listening)* He's saying "You have to have an abortion. I'll take you to the clinic tomorrow and you're going to get this taken care of."

(Rachel suddenly stops talking. She lies completely still.)

Rachel. . . breathe. You are safe. You are re-experiencing this only to

Jyoti Ma • 133

learn from it. Be there now, and tell me what you're feeling.

R: I'm so scared. I'm so scared I can't move. *(Now barely a whisper)* My grandfather wants to kill me. He wants me to die. He doesn't want me.

(And then she snaps back into the first experience, when she was 16)

R: But, I got to live. . . I got to live. . . but I. . . killed my baby. My baby didn't get to live. . . What have I done? *(The deep sounds of pain that come from her are beyond conscious understanding or description)*

R: I don't deserve to live. I don't deserve to be happy. I deserve to suffer and to be in darkness.

The pain of these two experiences ran so deeply it took many sessions to completely heal. In time, Rachel has learned to release the pain of these experiences and to embrace love, healing, and peace. When we first began, Rachel's conscious mind held no understanding of the pain she was in or even the fact she had negative feelings about having an abortion. But her soul was damaged in a real and terrible way from both her experience in the womb and her later decision to abort the baby within her own womb. On the deepest level, a part of her soul was living in an indescribable hell and the pain and self-loathing was slowly leaking out to poison every aspect of her life.

....

Jeff, age 54, came in desperate for help. He shared with me that he has had an ideal life, in all the ways he can imagine. He had two loving parents and supportive grandparents. He has always been surrounded by individuals who love him, including siblings, friends, and extended family. His family was blessed with financial security and his father had always been able to support them, fulfilling both needs and wants. He excelled academically and received a good education. He has been married for 25 years and has five children whom he loves and who love him.

I listened as he expressed these things about his life and then gently asked, "Why are you here?"

His response came in a shaking voice: "I live in Hell. Every day I am in emotional and physical pain. I feel like I have been ripped to pieces and am scattered throughout the universe. I don't know how to express to you what I'm feeling, but I hate everything about myself. I hate myself so much. I feel so worthless. *I hurt on every level all the time.* No matter how hard I try to do everything right and to focus on the incredible blessings within my life, all I feel is pain and unworthiness. I cannot find any rational explanation for how I feel."

We were unable to connect Jeff with any positive resources in the beginning of the session. All attempts to try to connect with his Highest Self and with God seemed to be blocked. I felt led to guide him directly to the source of the pain and negative emotion he was feeling. I still cry even now, each time I think of this experience.

....

(Jeff is in the womb, but not within his mother from this lifetime. He has regressed to a separate life experience and the doctor is in the process of performing an abortion)

Jeff, what core emotions are you feeling?

J: *(He's lost in his own experience and doesn't seem to hear me)* They don't want me! They don't want me and I have to go back! Oh, please God, please no. Please stop. *(Sobbing now from the depth of his soul- more intense than anything I have ever heard before)* STOP! STOP! NO! No No No! *(Screaming now. Screaming at the top of his lungs as his body is jerking and twisting in every direction. It's obvious he is in incredibly intense pain. His body is moving in completely unnatural movements and directions. I want to pull him from the memory but am prompted to wait. I cry silently as I watch him continue. Screaming. Twisting. Jerking. Sobbing. And then he is still.)*

(I wait several minutes before gently asking) **What is happening?**

J: They killed me. They tore me apart. My body is dead. *(Long pause)* They didn't want me.

(Without any prompting he continues)

J: I'm worthless. I'm unwanted.

Jeff, what did you lose here?

J: *(With the deepest sadness you can possibly imagine)* Everything. My soul is broken. I have nothing left but a tiny sliver. This tiny sliver of myself is all that came with me into my new life. Everything else within me is darkness and pain.

It took many sessions and much time before we were able to find, heal, and reconnect Jeff with the lost parts of himself. He still has much work to do. The pain and brokenness was beyond description. But, with love and light, all healing is possible. He has found new hope in that truth and he holds onto that sliver of hope to give him strength as he continues to move forward in his healing journey.

Chapter Twelve

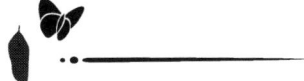

Destructive Patterns

*"Negative patterns will repeat throughout
our existence, unless we decide to jump off the wheel
and create a new path."*

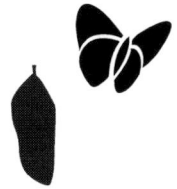

I hope it's becoming clear that our reality is greatly shaped by our experiences and expectations. When we believe something, it's what we attract and also what we see. When these beliefs and expectations are negative and dark, the effect in our life is painful and destructive. When we learn to release negative energy and to heal the misunderstandings and false conclusions, we help to create a happier and more fulfilling life and we can end the cycle of repeating negative experiences.

It's important to keep in mind so I'll say it again, negative conclusions and false beliefs are often the result of misunderstanding and limited information. We may conclude something that is completely erroneous, but regardless, once it's settled into our subconscious and a broken little piece of our soul believes it, it begins to affect our life story.

Any time we are triggered in an emotional way or experience any level of stress, our fight or flight reflex kicks in. When the blood rushes from the brain and into the extremities, our broken fragments and inner child take hold of the reigns and function in the best way they know how. Unfortunately, these parts of ourselves are making decisions with limited understanding and a whole lot of false beliefs. The result is a person who acts out in emotion, rage, addiction, or behaviors that seem completely irrational later when the calmer and wiser self takes back control.

Beliefs about the world as well as beliefs about our self play out in many different ways. Clients are often surprised when they come in wanting help with a current life situation or relationship and once in trance find themselves back in an early time or situation they would have never consciously connected to the current issue.

Heart-Centered Hypnotherapy literally gets to the "heart" of the matter. And this heart is where the healing must take place in order for positive changes to truly be lasting.

As we find and heal these hurting, broken, and misinformed pieces of our self, we become more aligned with our truest self- our Highest Self. As we heal, this Highest Self can better guide us in creating our healthiest and happiest existence. We begin to feel whole again, rather than broken, scattered, empty, and torn.

When we operate based on love and truth, rather than misunderstanding and lies, every area of our life gets better by leaps and bounds.

SUSAN, age 29, is a physically healthy and active adult. She has been involved in a variety of community service opportunities throughout her life and holds a supervisory position at her place of employment. Her husband of two years has a daughter from a previous marriage. She has an active social and professional life. Despite her greatest efforts, she never feels as though she belongs in any group. Upon external observation, one would likely consider her a confident, enjoyable, and well liked individual. However, internally she is bombarded by constant feelings of being rejected and left out. She cannot recall being part of any group to which she felt fully included and accepted. After years of feeling this way, she decided to seek help in understanding these emotions.

She struggled to relax enough to go into hypnosis. Once in trance she would pull in and out, afraid of letting go and trusting me to take care of her. With some practice and encouragement we were finally able to create an environment where she was able to fully relax and access her subconscious mind.

Go to a recent situation where you felt left out and abandoned. Tell me what's happening.

S: I'm on the phone with my husband. He and his daughter went to buy a new bicycle together. He's telling me about taking her on a ride. *(She stops talking. A tear starts to drip slowly down each of her cheeks. Her lips purse together to try to hide the sadness)*

What are you feeling? It's okay to feel whatever it is you're feeling; you're doing well. You are safe to express yourself.

S: I'm pretending to be happy for them. I'm telling him it's great they got to do that together. . .I hate it. I hate that they are doing things together and bonding and I'm not there. They don't care that I'm not there. *(Her voice sounding tired and defeated)* They should want me there. I'm so tired of being left out.

Where are you feeling this emotion, this sadness at being left out?

S: I feel constricted. My throat is closing off. I am HURTING! *(She is holding one hand on her throat and the other on her upper abdomen)*

Tell him everything you want to say. Speak it aloud and don't try to filter.

S: *(With anger and frustration)* I don't want to be left out! I don't deserve this! I'm sick and tired of pretending. I hate this. You should care that I'm not there! You should treat me like I matter. I hate this stupid fake enthusiasm! I HURT TOO! I AM HURTING! I am amazing. Why can't you see it? I deserve to be a part of the family! I deserve to be loved too! *(The anger breaking back into sadness as she now whispers)* I am so tired of hurting; so tired of being left out.

Focus on those feelings, hurting and being left out. Take yourself to the source of that emotion. Let yourself travel to the first time you felt hurt and left out.

S: I'm little. I don't know how old but I'm looking at three pictures on the wall. Me and my two brothers. We look the same. We are each beautiful. But they are loved and I am not. My grandmother loves them but she doesn't love me. *(She's holding her abdomen again and begins to sob)*

Tell your grandmother everything you want to say. Express to her how this makes you feel.

S: Grammy it's so unfair. You hate me. You hate me and I can't do anything about it. I have your hands, don't you see? Don't you see I'm just as special as Kaden? You hate my mom and so you hate me. I want you to love me. You favor my brothers. You let them do everything. I can't do anything. You play with them and help them and include them. I get left out. You tell me No. You stop me from being included. *(And now yelling with sorrow and anger)* It is so unfair! You are my grandmother! Why don't you love me? LOVE ME! Include me! Let me be a part of you. *(Anger is gone, only the sadness remains)* Please, Grammy. Please.

We spent more time in hypnosis, visiting different times in Susan's life to help her see the pattern this early emotion and experience had created. In grade school, on the playground, at girls camp, in high school clubs, in employment, and even now, in her marriage she continued the pattern of feeling left out and hurt. Once she recognized the source of these emotions and gained this awareness we were able to go through energy release and healing exercises. Her new and healthier decision is now:

I'm included. I'm enough. I'm OK alone. Even when I'm not there, I'm still loved. I'm still included.

Lisa, age 39, began hypnotherapy in hopes of understanding why everything in her life seems to be failing. She owns a small business; it was thriving but is now rapidly declining in sales and profit. It took several sessions before she was ready and able to go this deeply into the pain and to receive this self-insight.

In your last session you came to understand a subconscious belief you hold about your life. We are going to explore that further today, to help you understand where it came from and to help guide you in letting it go. "What brings me joy, brings me pain." I invite you to simply breathe and focus on this belief. Allow yourself to be taken to the source. Easily and effortlessly follow this belief back to the source. *(Within a few minutes it's apparent that she has found her way back to another time in her life. She is lying still. It looks as though she is petrified, afraid to move)* **Lisa, when you're ready, please tell me where you are.**

L: *(It takes her several minutes before responding. Her words come out in a whisper, barely discernible)* I'm camping. There's a man here. *(She begins sobbing now, but silently. As though she's afraid to make a sound but can no longer hold back her tears. She's shaking intensely but trying to lie still)* I was asleep. I thought it was my husband. This man broke into my tent and he's doing things to me. *(She can't speak anymore as the tears and the shaking are too intense)*

Lisa, we're going to leave this place now. I want you to feel your resources with you now. Remember your wise adult self? Feel her with you and ask her to give you the strength to get up and leave now. Allow her to guide you somewhere safe and tell me when you're there.

L: I'm next to the ocean. The man isn't here. I'm safe.

I would like you to express to me some of what you're feeling after witnessing this experience again.

L: I'm confused and scared. I feel so guilty.

What is the guilt about?

L: I was enjoying it. *(Tears and the energy of remorse are fully present)* I thought it was my husband. I was asleep. Why didn't I know? Why didn't I stop him? I'm bad. I'm a bad person. Even when I realized it wasn't my husband I was too afraid. I couldn't move. I couldn't speak. I was so scared and I didn't know what to do. I just laid there.

And as a result of this experience, what conclusions have you made about yourself or about your life?

L: I can't trust myself because I don't know what I'm doing. It's unsafe to feel joy. My joy comes with negative consequences. What brings me joy, brings me pain.

How is this continuing to affect your life now?

L: I'm afraid when things go well. I'm afraid to be happy. When anything has the potential to bring joy, I need it to stop. It's not safe. I can't trust myself. I don't know what I'm doing.

(We pause at this point to allow for negative energy release and balancing. We begin the process of extinguishing the negative emotions and false beliefs. We call in all available loving sources to be with her as she begins the healing process. With time, she was able to express the following)

L: I can reclaim my power and learn to trust myself again. As I take time to care for myself, I will find balance and peace. As I forgive myself, I will again find the ability to feel joy and will uncover my creativity. I need to take time to be present, to laugh, and to let myself be who I am. Trust. Faith. Faith in God and faith in myself. It's all going to be OK.

(After two more sessions, Lisa received enough healing to be able to claim the following affirmations)

L: I am happy, healthy, wealthy, beautiful, and wise. I trust that I am divinely led. My joy creates joy for those around me. The success of my business creates more freedom for my family. I choose to live my life in the present moment, free of the pain of the past and enjoying the beauty around me.

Braden, age 9, is a playful and physically healthy child. He does well academically and has a good group of friends. However; he struggles emotionally, often being described as "overly dramatic" and "intensely sensitive". He is fiercely competitive, especially toward his brother who is 18 months younger than he is. In school and social settings he frequently collapses to the ground in tears if he makes a mistake or if things don't play out as well as he has planned for them to in his mind. Winning at everything is extremely important to him. His mother brought him to the session seeking to understand why he struggles with these emotional tendencies and hoping to find a way to begin helping him feel more secure and balanced.

It looks as though you are feeling uncomfortable. Tell me what you're experiencing.

B: I'm angry. And really really sad. *(He has tears forming and is clutching his hands together and holding them at the center of his chest)*

Hold onto those feelings Braden and go to a recent time you felt them. When you get there, please tell me about it.

B: David wants an apple just because I want an apple. He does everything I do. He copies me. I feel angry. *(Pause)* And really sad. I don't want him to copy me.

I want you to go to another time you felt these emotions; where you felt hurt and sad.

B: I was beating David at a race. I'm seven, he's five and he jumped on me and bit me right in the back. I'm really angry. And I'm mad that he caught me. And it really hurts. He hurts me. He hurts me and I get in trouble. I needed to win that race. *(His body is twisting as he is re-experiencing this pain)*

You're doing so well Braden. I'm very proud of you. I would like you to go back again, back to the first time you felt really sad and hurt.

B: *(His countenance becomes visibly younger. He has twisted his body into a side lying fetal position and is clinging very tightly to his knees)* I'm three. David is one. He's getting lots of attention. Everyone likes him. Everyone thinks he is so cute and fun. They don't talk to me very much. They tickle him and sing to him and tell him how sweet he is. (Pause) I hit him. *(Remorse and sadness fill his body and are coming out through his tears)* I just hit him a little bit but Grandpa says I should get whipped. He wants mom to whip me with a hickory switch. I'm so sad. I am so angry. I don't want a brother. I'm so mad I have a brother. Maybe if I didn't have a brother, people would like me too.

Braden, at this time you made a conclusion about yourself. What is it?

B: Maybe David is better than me. I need to be different. *(Tears are flowing freely and he's gently rocking his body)*

We visited a few more experiences to allow Braden to fully recognize this pattern in his life of feeling less than his brother and needing to prove himself. After several re-lived experiences and some very intense energy release, Braden was ready to let go of the old conclusion he drew. He chose to invite his highest power, Jesus, into his safe and relaxing place in his mind to help him draw a new conclusion.

B: Jesus just told me I'm awesome, cool, funny, smart, and fantastic. *(His smile is huge and his body lying in complete peace and comfort, literally radiating light)* I AM FANTASTIC!

Chapter Thirteen

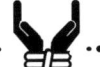

Energetic Bonds

*"Carrying the darkness of another will keep
both of you out of the Light."*

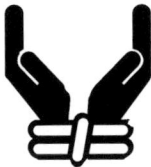

We exist on many levels and are multidimensional beings. We can connect with others emotionally and physically, but we also connect energetically. Some people we feel drawn to. Others we feel intensely aversive to. Some people we love and feel truly connected to. Others seem to have an unseen power over us even when we may try to break away.

Energetic bonds can be both positive and negative. If we share an energy bond of love with our spouse, loving energy and positive messages can flow easily from one heart to the other. Energetic bonds can be healing and helpful. They can connect us in beautiful and powerful ways, allowing us to truly tune into and understand those we love.

When they are positive, these bonds can serve our highest good and bless our relationships. But when they are negative, these energetic bonds can be incredibly destructive. It's very common for those who have been in abusive or dominant relationships to have energetic bonds, or cords, connecting them to their abuser. These cords allow the dark energy from the abuser to continue tugging, pulling, and manipulating the individual. These negative bonds may also be created by an overbearing and controlling mother, father, or other authority figure. They subconsciously send out a cord of energy to cling to the other individual. These negative bonds make it difficult to completely pull away and make choices independently.

Through Heart-Centered Hypnotherapy these energetic bonds can be identified. Negative bonds can be removed and positive bonds created or strengthened; allowing individuals to experience greater personal freedom and to think more clearly.

These energetic bonds can also be created between deceased loved ones and those they've left behind. When a person dies, their spirit has a few options. No one is forced to go into the light and to continue progressing. Some choose to linger. They often linger out of fear or negative emotions. But other times, they linger out of love. They don't want to leave those they care about. The problem is, unless the person who has died chooses to go to the light and be fully cleansed and healed of the weight and burden they've carried from their lifetime, they inadvertently share the burden and darkness with those still living. I refer to these spirits as earthbound. They are not necessarily evil or bad and many even have good intention, but they are also not filled with light.

If it's apparent that an earthbound spirit is lingering and affecting a client, I encourage the spirit to move into the light first and then to come back to help as a positive influence when it can. Clients in a trance are often able to see, sense, and communicate directly with these spirits. I guide them in knowing what to say and how to encourage the spirits to move forward.

Even out of trance, you can begin to consciously pay attention to the energy around you and within your environment. Shifts in temperature, attitude, increased levels of contention, or even a general feeling of uneasiness can often rightly be attributed to the presence of an earthbound spirit. You may speak to them directly, even though unseen, and remind them to look within for their divine light. They can also be instructed to look up; angels are often hovering and waiting to help them.

If you have loved ones who are dying, give them permission to leave and encourage them to move into the light for healing and growth. Reassure them that you will be better off if they make the choice to go, and to only return to watch over you once they have spent time in the light.

Smudging, a Native American ritual involving the burning of white sage, is also an effective way to clear negative energy and spirits from a person or space. I have an introductory class about smudging on my website that I encourage you to consider. It's a process I use regularly within my home and office space and the difference it makes is palpable. My children often come home from school feeling down and ask me to "do that smoke thing" to help them feel better.

I will share a few experiences to illustrate these concepts. Holding pieces of someone else's energy, giving pieces of our own energy away, having negative bonds and cords, and being attached to earthbound spirits are all very common occurrences. In the beginning it caught me by surprise and honestly rather blew my mind. But now, it's just another day in the office!

Note: Not all Heart-Centered Hypnotherapists work directly with clearing spirits and other energies. There are various levels of structured Heart-Centered Hypnotherapy training. Some learning and skill comes only with experience.

....

Sally, age 22, recently separated from her boyfriend. They have one child together, a boy, who is now 4 years old.

....

Sally, where are you?

S: A few days ago Jack and I got into a fight. He texted me and asked if I was upset and I didn't respond. I always avoid contention. It's easier to just ignore things.

By ignoring that text you chose to bury your feelings. Feel into your body now and find the feelings you buried. Breathe into your body and simply feel where in your body is tight or tense. *(She nods and places her hands on her abdomen)* **Now, Sally, speak the words that didn't get spoken. Tell Jack the feelings and words you held back.**

S: *(Her face begins to flush and her fists clench. It's apparent that she's feeling very angry. When she speaks her voice is seething)* Jack, you make me feel like I'm the only one who messes up. You make me feel like I'm a bad person. I hate it. I hate you for it. I hate everything about this situation. I can't stand feeling this way. Of course I'm upset! You go out of your way to hurt me and say things that you know will cut me to the very core. Why? I don't understand. I try to be who you want me to be and yet it's never been good enough. I'm done! I'm so done! Let me be. Let me go. Stop pretending that you're perfect. Not everything is my fault. *(The anger is gone now. Tears begin to form as the energy of anger is replaced by sadness)*

Sally, it's been six months since you and Jack split and yet it appears that he still has quite an emotional hold on you. I would like you to check your body now. Feel, sense, and look for anything attaching you to Jack. It might be a cord, or chain. . .

S: *(She cuts me off)* It's a rope. It's thick, braided, and gray. It's coming out of my spine. It feels like he is holding it in his hands and jerking me around. It's holding me back. He's manipulating and controlling me with it.

It's very common for us to develop negative bonds such as this with individuals who have played such a major role in our lives. This rope keeps you connected to Jack in a way that hurts both of you. Negative bonds are never in our best interest. Would you like to release it?

S: It's like he still needs me. He thinks he needs me. But it's not healthy. And, I'm so used to relying on him for emotional support. I don't know if I am strong enough to do it on my own. I don't know if I can release the cord.

I don't want you to try to release it until you feel ready. I'm going to play a song and move some energy for you. While I do so I also ask that any and all loved ones or angels who are willing to support you, to join you now and help you see or sense their presence in some way. Allow them to teach, help, support, or heal you in any way that serves your highest good. *(During the song she cries a steady stream of tears. Her demeanor also begins to change from one of hopelessness and despair to a stronger, more light filled countenance with an energy of peace surrounding her)*

Who has chosen to be with you today to show their support and offer you assistance in your session?

S: There are so many. I feel angels all around me. *(A quiet voice of respect and awe has replaced the anger, tension, and sadness)*

Is there anyone with you whom you recognize?

S: Yes. I feel my Heavenly Father. I see Jesus Christ. I can't believe they're here. I sense my Highest Self and my family. I even see my sisters who have passed on. They've all come to support me. I feel their love so strongly. *(Now choking back tears of joy and relief)*

What are they helping you to know?

S: Even though it's scary, it's not helping anybody. I gave Jack this rope to control me because I believed he could do a better job than I can of guiding my life. But I was wrong. It's not his place. And he's too full of darkness. If I believe in myself and rely on healthy relationships it will be better for all of us. I can release the rope and end the negative attachment to Jack.

Do you feel ready to do so?

S: Yes. I feel so supported and loved. I believe I am ready.

Invite your angels and loved ones to help you. They will know how to guide you in releasing this negative bond and healing from its effects. (I play another song and continue to do energy healing techniques as she experiences her process of release)

S: It's done. *(A huge smile spreads across her face)* Jesus helped me remove the rope and replaced the missing pieces of my backbone. He replaced fear with courage. He also gave me the knowledge that the power He can give me is so much greater than anything else I could ever have or long for.

That's beautiful Sally. Tell me specifically the things you are reclaiming now that this rope has been removed and this healing has taken place.

S: I am reclaiming my ability to stand up for myself in a way that's kind but also stops others from walking all over me. I am also reclaiming happiness and self-confidence.

Sally, I feel there may be a message coming. Please simply breathe and allow any message to come into your mind.

S: *(After a pause and gentle breathing)* It's from God. He wants me to know I am learning important things. I can continue to have faith. Things will continue to work out. I can release the fear little bit by little bit. I'm deserving of help and I have many people who love and support me. *(She pauses again and laughs)* He really wants me to understand that I don't have to be perfect.

I'd like to invite your Highest Self to help you choose a new guiding affirmation for your life, something to replace the old lies and fears.

S: I believe in my ability to take my life in a positive direction. I am worthy of love and happiness. I allow God and my loved ones to support and help me as I learn, heal, and grow stronger each day.

Jennifer, age 32, is a stay at home mother. In a previous session she discovered a close tie of binge eating to underlying emotions of loneliness and sadness. These are emotions she was not consciously aware of until that session. Once identified, she has been able to recognize the negative influence of these suppressed emotions. She now desires to understand where they are coming from and how to overcome them.

Jennifer, I want you to focus intently on the emotions of sadness and loneliness. Go to the most recent time you felt these feelings intensely and tell me about it.

J: I am at home. My husband has been gone for several days. The kids are asleep and the house is so quiet. I feel really empty. Someone else should be here. *(She quietly begins to cry; eyes closed and dripping silent tears)*

Focus on that Jennifer. Focus on "Someone else should be here." What emotion is behind that?

J: Sorrow. Loneliness.

We are going to go further back now. Allow yourself to drop into one of the first times you felt these intense feelings of sorrow and loneliness. Go to the source of these emotions.

J: It's Christmas eve. Well, early Christmas morning I guess. I'm bleeding. I am having a miscarriage. *(The silent tears are steadily flowing now and there is a long pause as she is reliving this experience.)* The ultra sound tech is here. He's talking to the nurse about what a great paycheck this is going to bring him; double pay for the holiday plus time and a half for coming in during the night. *(The tears are no longer silent. Her breathing is rapid and she's gasping in-between sobs)* He just informed me that there is no sign of the baby. It's gone. *(Her tears suddenly stop and there is no further sign of emotion)*

Jennifer, you've buried your emotions again. It's time to face them instead. Drop back into this experience and allow yourself to become aware of all you are feeling. Do not block these emotions. This is a safe and appropriate time to feel them. Speak what you need to as we do the energy release exercise.

J: *(Barely a whisper)* I'm so sorry. I'm so sorry I didn't grieve for you. I went to work that morning and acted like nothing was wrong. *(The tears are flowing again and her voice is rising)* It's my fault! I shouldn't have lifted that table. I felt you die inside of me! I felt you die! I knew better and I did it anyway! *(Screaming at the top of her lungs)* Why am I so stupid? Why do I always have to prove that I'm invincible? I killed my baby! I killed you!

(After several minutes of energy release, sobbing, and further dialogue, Jennifer collapses onto the floor and lays her head into her knees. The negative energy is released and she is simply allowing herself to rest and be fully in tune with herself and this moment. Then, without prompting of any sort, she relays the following)

J: He's here. My baby is here. His name is Matthew. *(A full and beautiful smile crosses her face and her tears become tears of joy)* He wants me to know it's not my fault. That he loves me. That he's never left me. He wants me to be happy. *(Then, she speaks directly to her child)* Matthew, have you been to the light? *(Pauses)* I want you to go with Jesus and be healed of the sadness you've had to carry because of me. I will be OK now. When you are healed and full of light, please come back and be with me and our family as often as you are able to. But don't linger here in darkness any longer. We can love each other now. I know about you now and I know why I've been lonely. But now that I know about you, I don't have to be lonely anymore. *(She again speaks to the hypnotherapist)* He's gone now. But he will be back. I

Jyoti Ma • 159

never realized his little spirit was still with me. He was trying to hold all the sadness for me and protect me. We can both heal now. I feel a warm light surrounding me, holding me. We're both going to be OK.

After three months, Jennifer reported that Matthew returned to be with her. He is now able to be a positive part of her life. She does not see him but senses when he is present and at times even receives quiet messages from him directly into her heart and mind. She says "He asked me this past Mother's Day to acknowledge him when people ask me how many children I have. It's important to him that he is included and that others know of his existence. My husband has felt his presence on more than one occasion now as well and we cannot wait until one day we will meet him when our time on this Earth is done. The feeling that someone is missing and the overwhelming sorrow is gone; it's been replaced by feelings of peace and happiness."

Patrick, age 38, has been short tempered and angry with others for little to no reason. He expressed that he struggles to accept any compliments and feels they are empty words. He is also disappointed and annoyed with the principle at the school where he teaches.

Feel, sense, and see your safe and relaxing place. Begin to invite your Highest Self to appear. I invite him to appear in any form you might recognize and connect with.

P: I see him as a man. He's so carefree. He's even laughing and dancing around in the sunlight. *(A half smile creeps onto his face, a glimmer of hope that this part of him exists)* He has the joy and love that I seek. He's fun. He's Light- he enjoys keeping things light. He really enjoys life. He's giggling as I watch him. *(He laughs out loud now as he expresses to me what he's seeing)*

As you watch him, what are you feeling?

P: Relief. I feel relieved that he's happy, not angry or sad. I feel peace that he's inside of me somewhere. I feel some hope that maybe I can find a way to unlock him, and let him into my life.

We're going to move back into the negative feelings now, the ones you were feeling when we talked before. Find anger and disappointment in your body again. Allow these feelings to come up and notice where the energy concentrates in your body.

P: *(He places his hands on his stomach)* It's right here. It's so tight. It feels like knives twisting and turning inside.

I invite you to speak for your stomach. Speak the words and feelings that are being held there. The words will simply come,

there is nothing you need to do but open your mouth and give them permission to flow.

P: I'm so angry. *(His voice begins to rise) I am so angry! (Shouting now)* I am angry that I have things to say and people aren't listening. I am so mad that people aren't doing what they are supposed to do. They offer false praise. Everything is fake. People are fake.

There is someone specific coming to mind. Notice who it is and speak to them directly.

P: Carmen, you aren't being honest. Your words mean nothing. *(Yelling again)* You feed us crap. You don't have any idea what kind of teacher I am, you aren't paying attention. You speak words of praise but they are empty. You are not doing your job! You let us down. . . You let me down. You never apologize for it. *(His yelling dies down but there is cracking in his voice)* I feel so annoyed. Don't tell me I'm doing something well if you don't know what I'm doing. You are supposed to be my leader. I need you to lead me. *(Even quieter now)* Please, I need you to see me, know me, and lead me.

We're going to bring those feelings back up now. Breathe back into the feelings of anger, mixed with sadness. Allow them to come back up and we'll follow them back now. *(I help these feelings increase and then guide him back to an earlier time)* **Where are you now, Patrick?**

P: I'm in school. I'm a child. There's a teacher who is talking to me in the hallway. He's telling me I'm special. He's saying I did well on the testing and that I am gifted. I feel confused. *(He pauses and then continues with tears beginning to form)* There is nothing special about how I process information. I am not special. He's wrong. He's lying to me but I don't know why he's even saying these things. I feel very confused.

Your belief about not being special, it feels like it was already in place before this moment. Is that true? *(He nods)* **I'd like you to go back to that moment, when you decided you were not special. Follow your breath and let me know when you get there.**

P: I'm in my childhood home, in the basement. It's dark. The basement here was so scary. It always felt yucky, dark, like something was there that didn't belong.

And what are you feeling here right now. Be back in this place, back in this childhood moment.

P: I feel sad. I feel unimportant. I feel like there is nothing about me that is good, that I am not special. And I feel really angry. *(His voice rises as he speaks about the anger)*

Breathe into these emotions and tell me which one feels the strongest right now.

P: Anger. It's really strong. But *(pauses)* it doesn't feel like it's mine.

Good Patrick, you're becoming aware. Breathe into that anger again and feel how it's separate from you, how it's different than your own energy. I'm going to ask you a few questions. Your Highest Self knows the answers so simply allow those answers to come into your mind. Does this energy belong to you?

P: No. It doesn't.

Does it belong to another person from your life, a friend or family member?

P: No. It doesn't.

Does it seem to have a mind of its own?

P: Yes. It definitely does.

Now that we've identified it as being separate from you and having a mind of its own, I'm going to speak to it directly. You can relate to me it's answers. Can you see this being?

P: It's very dark. I only see a dark shadow.

Now that we've identified you, you will not be allowed to stay. Why

Jyoti Ma • 163

are you here?

P: He's really mad; like, really mad. He's not at all happy that you're talking to him.

That's alright. I am not worried about or insulted by his anger. *(Speaking again to this other being)* I understand that you're angry. I know you're not happy that we've identified you. But, now that we have, you have two choices. The first choice is to go back to where you came from, to turn back to darkness and pain- to be lost and alone. This is not what we would want for you. But you may choose it.

P: He's still angry but he's listening.

I invite you to look inside yourself. Look past the anger, go deeper and tell me what you see.

P: Under the anger, there's a lot of sadness. *(Patrick begins to cry as he feels the weight of sorrow this being is carrying)* There's so much sadness.

The anger and sadness have been hiding your true self and your real value for a very long time. I invite you to look even deeper. Look under both the anger and sadness, look through the darkness deep within yourself and please tell me what you see.

P: *(With surprise)* There's a light. He sees a tiny flicker of light within himself.

This light is proof that you have a second choice. The second choice is to turn back to the light, to be restored to peace and wholeness. There is someone coming who would like to help you, if you make this choice. Look up and tell me who is coming.

P: My grandmother. *(He is now crying openly)* My grandmother is coming to help this spirit.

And now it's time to make a choice. Will you go with Patrick's grandmother to be taught and healed and restored to beauty and light?

P: Yes. Yes, he wants to go. My grandma is smiling, she's so glad.

Before he leaves we need to know in what ways he's been affecting you. *(Speaking again to the spirit)* Please, help Patrick see the influence you've been having on him and remove all lingering darkness you have placed within him. Take all of it with you into the light, that all of it might be healed and transformed.

P: He's removing doubt. He's pulling out the anger. I feel these really deep roots within me. I feel him pulling everything out by these deep roots. *(I play music and call on all loving sources to come to help Patrick begin to release the weight of darkness within him. He cries deeply as he feels loved ones and angels coming to his aide)*

Please tell me when you feel that he and all effects of him are gone.

P: He's gone. It's all gone. *(Pauses)* And, he says thank you. He's so excited to know that light and peace can exist for him. *(He pauses again)* But, this is weird, but I feel like I've lost a friend. I feel really empty and alone. *(Tears streaming)*

He's been with you a very long time. And although he was dark, he was filling a void within you. This void is still there and it's time to fill it with something that better serves you. We're going to move back to your safe place now, back to the beautiful place where you felt connected to your Highest Self. *(I help him find his way back and then go on)* Beside your Highest Self is the piece of yourself that was lost long ago, the part of you that broke off and created the void that the darkness then filled. Describe for me what you see or sense.

P: It's a young boy, an innocent young boy. *(He pauses as he comes to understand what he's seeing)* It's me as a young boy. It's the part of me that's innocent and beautiful; a part of me that knows my inner value and worth.

You'll know if it's the right time, so trust the answer that comes.

Patrick, is it the right time to invite this boy back? Would you like to help him find his place within yourself again?

P: *(With many tears and choking on his words)* Yes. I want him back.

Take him by the hands and look into his eyes. When you are ready, tell him "Welcome back". He will disappear as he re-enters your body and spirit. *(I play music and help move the energy to invite this lost soul piece back into his body, mind, and spirit)*

Patrick, what have you reclaimed today?

P: Today, I reclaim my joy for life. I reclaim my curiosity. I reclaim my ability to see my own value and to receive compliments with trust. I can now see brightness in others instead of darkness. I recognize that I can be loving when I feel frustrated. I am no longer influenced by anger, instead I choose to come from a place of love and innocence. I am me again.

Chapter Fourteen

It's Time to Heal

"There is no better time than today to reset your course and to align with Love."

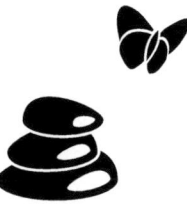

My spiritual name is Jyoti Ma. In translation this means, Mother of Light. When I received this name, it came with instruction that it is more than a title. It is my life path. Bringing others back to a knowledge of the Light and beauty within themselves is my purpose and calling. I have so much more of my own healing work to do. I am still broken, hurting, and have layers of darkness in various fragments within my soul. But I have begun. I am taking steps to heal. We do not need to be perfect in order to lift and help those around us. I am coming to understand this better each day. The Light I carry within myself can find the Light you carry and together we can shine our Light into the world. Light overcomes darkness. Light heals pain. Light guides us to where we desire to be. Light is Love, and Love is our truest purpose and identity.

By reading this book, you have already begun to crack and weaken the layers of darkness within yourself. Becoming aware is the first step to change. I invite you to begin pondering and inviting your Highest Self to open your eyes to see areas within you that may need help and healing. I created an online class to help support you in recognizing and strengthening the connection to your Highest Self. It's a beautiful place to start. You will then be in tune as your inner voice, your own Highest Self, guides you in the next steps of your personal healing journey. You may find this course on my website, www.healingforlifewa.com.

I also welcome you to connect with me on Facebook and YouTube where I regularly share inspirational messages, blog posts, and guided meditations designed to bring healing and positive change. You can find these links on my website as well. Melody Litton is my every day name and the one I've used with my classes and other books. But when I facilitate healing and tune into the soul of another, it's with the help of my Highest Self. To honor this part of myself and to acknowledge the gifts she brings me; this book has been published with the name Jyoti Ma.

There are many Heart-Centered Hypnotherapists who can walk with you as you heal. You may also be led to any variety of other healing modalities and practitioners with various skills and specialties. Trust the promptings that come and seek healing in the way that you know is right for you.

Decide today to be a little kinder; choose to see the hurting child inside the ones who offend you and also, inside of yourself. Respond to others with love, rather than anger. Lift those who try to tear you down.

Call on the Light when darkness seems overpowering. And never again forget: *You are a divine, radiant being with unlimited potential.*

Become a Heart-Centered Hypnotherapist

Change the world; one soul at a time

or

Find a provider to continue your personal healing journey

www.wellness-institute.org

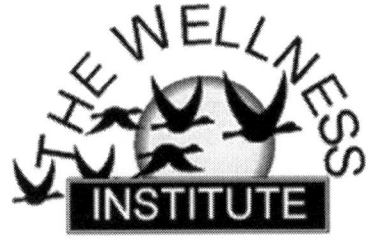

Connect with the author and learn more about her online classes and other books at

www.healingforlifewa.com

Made in the USA
Columbia, SC
18 May 2017